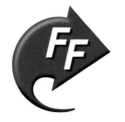

Chronic Obstructive Pulmonary Disease

..., MD FRCP

Professor of Respiratory and Environmental Medicine
ELEGI Colt Laboratories
University of Edinburgh Medical School, Edinburgh, UK

Stephen I Rennard MD

Larson Professor of Medicine
Pulmonary and Critical Care Medicine Section
Department of Internal Medicine
University of Nebraska Medical Center
Omaha, Nebraska, USA

HEALTH PRESS

Fast Facts – Chronic Obstructive Pulmonary Disease
First published March 2004
Reprinted December 2005

Text © 2004 William MacNee, Stephen I Rennard
© 2004 in this edition Health Press Limited
Health Press Limited, Elizabeth House, Queen Street, Abingdon,
Oxford OX14 3LN, UK
Tel: +44 (0)1235 523233
Fax: +44 (0)1235 523238

Book orders can be placed by telephone or via the website.
For regional distributors or to order via the website, please go to:
www.fastfacts.com
For telephone orders, please call 01752 202301 (UK), +44 1752 202301 (Europe),
1 800 247 6553 (USA, toll free) or +1 419 281 1802 (Americas).

Fast Facts is a trademark of Health Press Limited.

The publisher and the authors have made every effort to ensure the accuracy of this
book, but cannot accept responsibility for any errors or omissions.

For all drugs, please consult the product labeling approved in your country for
prescribing information.

Registered names, trademarks, etc. used in this book, even when not marked as such,
are not to be considered unprotected by law.

A CIP record for this title is available from the British Library.

ISBN 1-899541-99-3

MacNee, W (William)
Fast Facts – Chronic Obstructive Pulmonary Disease/
William MacNee, Stephen I Rennard

Typesetting and page layout by Zed, Oxford, UK.

Printed by Fine Print (Services) Ltd, Oxford, UK.

Printed with vegetable inks on fully biodegradable and
recyclable paper manufactured from sustainable forests.

444   001
Low emissions
during production

Low
chlorine

Sustainable
forests

Glossary of abbreviations

COPD: chronic obstructive pulmonary disease

CT: computed tomography

DLCO: diffusing capacity in the lung for carbon monoxide, carbon monoxide transfer factor (sometimes called TLCO in the UK)

ECG: electrocardiography

FEV_1: forced expiratory volume in 1 second

FVC: forced vital capacity (the total volume of air that can be exhaled from a maximum inhalation to a maximum exhalation)

GOLD: Global Initiative for Chronic Obstructive Lung Disease

HDU: high-dependency unit

HRCT: high-resolution computed tomography

ICU: intensive care unit

IPPV: intermittent positive-pressure ventilation

K_{CO}: carbon monoxide transfer coefficient ($DLCO/V_A$)

MRC: Medical Research Council (UK)

NHLBI: National Heart, Lung and Blood Institute (USA)

NIPPV: non-invasive intermittent positive-pressure ventilation

NOTT: nocturnal oxygen therapy trial

$PaCO_2$: partial pressure of carbon dioxide in arterial blood

PaO_2: partial pressure of oxygen in arterial blood

PEF: peak expiratory flow

SaO_2: percentage oxygen saturation of arterial blood

V_A: ventilated alveolar volume, or accessible lung volume

V_D: dead space

V_T: tidal volume

VC: vital capacity

Introduction

Chronic obstructive pulmonary disease (COPD) has not always elicited sympathetic interest from the medical community. In their groundbreaking monograph on the natural history of COPD, Fletcher and colleagues chose the following quote to emphasize the self-perpetuating attitude which has unfortunately inhibited the understanding and management of COPD.

> '...medicine has come a long way since 1925, when Williams, writing *Middle age and old age*, could confidently assert: "Chronic bronchitis with its accompanying emphysema is a disease on which a good deal of wholly unmerited sympathy is frequently wasted. It is a disease of the gluttonous, bibulous, otiose and obese and represents a well-deserved nemesis for these unlovely indulgences ... the majority of cases are undoubtedly due to surfeit and self-indulgence."'

Since the landmark study of Fletcher and Peto, great gains have been made in understanding the pathogenesis, physiology, clinical features and management of COPD. Cigarette smoking, itself now regarded as a disease, is the major risk factor. However, COPD also occurs in non-smokers, and individuals vary greatly in their susceptibility. Moreover, COPD is a heterogeneous collection of syndromes with overlapping manifestations. This has led to considerable variance in definitions, confounding epidemiologic and cross-national studies. The Global Initiative for Chronic Obstructive Lung Disease (GOLD) was recently implemented in order to provide some uniformity. GOLD defines COPD as: **'a disease state characterized by airflow limitation that is not fully reversible. The airflow limitation is usually both progressive and associated with an abnormal inflammatory response of the lungs to noxious particles or gases'.**

COPD was estimated to be the twelfth leading cause of morbidity and the sixth leading cause of death worldwide in 1990. Of all the major diseases, COPD is the one for which the burden is increasing fastest. By 2020, COPD is expected to be the fifth leading cause of disability and the third leading cause of death (Figure 1). COPD

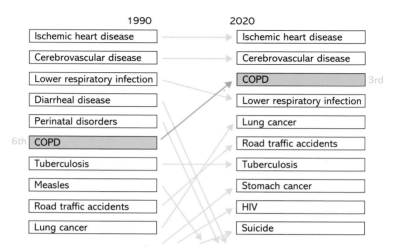

Figure 1 Predicted changes in global causes of mortality. Data from Murray and Lopez 1997.

patients, moreover, often make few complaints despite suffering considerable disability. As a result, although COPD can easily be diagnosed, it frequently is not.

The relationship between asthma and COPD has been particularly troublesome. Defining asthma as 'reversible' led to the inference that COPD is 'irreversible' and, therefore, that there was nothing to 'reverse' with treatment. Such a belief has served only to exacerbate the underdiagnosis and undermanagement of COPD patients. It is now recognized that COPD may be partially reversible and that there may be considerable overlap in the pathophysiological mechanisms that underlie asthma and the syndromes comprising COPD. Furthermore, some patients with asthma may develop COPD. The diagnostic problem, therefore, is not whether a patient has asthma *or* COPD, but rather whether *either* asthma or COPD is present, or both.

COPD is a very expensive disorder. Costs in the USA are estimated at nearly $32 billion annually; two thirds of these costs are direct and one third indirect. Since COPD is significantly underdiagnosed, these estimates are likely to be highly conservative.

Most costs associated with COPD are due to exacerbations, particularly those that result in hospitalization. Since exacerbations increase in frequency and require a greater level of care as COPD progresses, most costs are incurred in more severe cases as patients the end stage of the disease. Previous guidelines have emphasized treatment for patients who have lost half or two thirds of their lung function. Recent guidelines, however, recognize that diagnosis and treatment of COPD at earlier stages can offer significant benefits for the patient.

Currently available treatments, while unable to cure COPD, can offer considerable benefit by reducing symptoms, improving function and reducing exacerbations, and may decrease healthcare costs associated with COPD. This book is designed to present an up-to-date summary of our understanding of COPD and of how patients should be evaluated and managed.

Key references

Fletcher C, Peto R, Tinker C, Speizer FE. *The Natural History of Chronic Bronchitis and Emphysema: An Eight-Year Study of Early Chronic Obstructive Lung Disease in Working Men in London.* New York: Oxford University Press, 1976:1–272.

Fletcher C, Peto R. The natural history of chronic airflow obstruction. *BMJ* 1977;1:1645–8.

Global Initiative for Chronic Obstructive Lung Disease. *Global Strategy for the Diagnosis, Management, and Prevention of Chronic Obstructive Pulmonary Disease. NHLBI/WHO Workshop Report.* National Heart, Lung, and Blood Institute (USA), World Health Organization: 2001, updated 2003. www.goldcopd.com

Murray CJ, Lopez AD. Alternative projections of mortality and disability by cause 1990–2020: Global Burden of Disease Study. *Lancet* 1997;349:1498–1504.

Piquette CA, Rennard SI, Snider GL. Chronic bronchitis and emphysema. In: Murray JF, Nadel JA, eds. *Textbook of Respiratory Medicine,* 3rd edn. Philadelphia: WB Saunders, 2000:1187–1245.

In COPD, pathological changes occur in the central conducting airways, the peripheral airways, the lung parenchyma and the pulmonary vasculature. Inflammation induced by cigarette smoke underlies most pathological lesions associated with COPD. Inflammation also contributes to recurrent exacerbations of COPD, in which acute inflammation is superimposed on the chronic disease. There is now good evidence that all smokers develop lung inflammation; however, some individuals are more susceptible to the effects of cigarette smoke and are more severely affected. The extent of the pathological changes in the different lung compartments varies between individuals and results in the clinical and pathophysiological heterogeneity seen in patients with COPD.

Some believe that chronic asthma should be included as part of the spectrum of COPD. Although the clinical and physiological presentation of chronic asthma may be indistinguishable from that of COPD, the pathological changes are distinct from those in the majority of COPD cases due to cigarette smoking. Histologic features of COPD in the 15–20% of COPD patients who are non-smokers have not yet been studied.

Chronic bronchitis

Chronic bronchitis is defined clinically by the American Thoracic Society and the UK Medical Research Council as: '**the production of sputum on most days for at least three months in at least two consecutive years**'. This chronic hypersecretion of mucus results from changes in the central airways – the trachea, bronchi and bronchioles > 2–4 mm in internal diameter. Mucus is produced by mucus glands, which are present mainly in the larger airways, and by goblet cells, found in the airway epithelium. Hypertrophy of mucus glands occurs mainly in the larger bronchi, is evenly distributed throughout the lungs and is associated with infiltration of the glands by inflammatory cells (Figure 1.1). Mucus gland hypertrophy can be quantified by the Reid

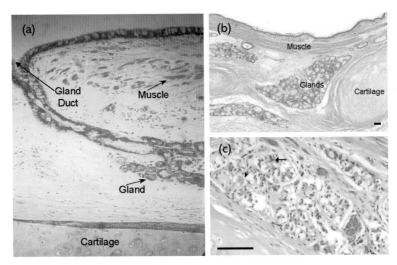

Figure 1.1 Pathological changes of the central airways in COPD. (a) A central bronchus from the lungs of a cigarette smoker with normal function shows small amounts of muscle present in subepithelium and small epithelial glands. (b) In a patient with chronic bronchitis the muscle appears as a thick bundle and the bronchial glands are enlarged. (c) At a higher magnification, these glands show evidence of a chronic inflammatory process involving polymorphonuclear leukocytes (arrowhead) and mononuclear cells, including plasma cells (arrow). Reproduced from the GOLD Workshop Report with the kind permission of Professor James C Hogg.

index, which is the ratio of the distance between the basement membrane of the airway epithelium and the cartilage to the thickness of the gland layer, and is normally 3:1. Alternatively, mucus gland size can be assessed by measurement of the absolute gland area, whereby the proportion of the wall occupied by glands is assessed. The volume of sputum production correlates better with mucus gland area or volume than with the Reid index. Sputum volume also correlates with the degree of inflammation in the airway wall, indicating the importance of abnormal regulation of secretions. In healthy never-smokers, goblet cells make up 10% of the columnar epithelial cells in the proximal airways and decrease in number in more distal airways, normally being absent in the terminal or respiratory bronchioles. By contrast, in smokers, goblet cells are not only present in increased numbers but also extend more peripherally. Metaplastic or dysplastic changes in the surface epithelium may replace the goblet cells of the normal respiratory epithelium in some smokers and hence may reduce the number of goblet cells in the proximal airways. The clinical significance of these varied anatomic alterations is unknown.

Recent studies using bronchoscopy to obtain lavage and biopsy samples have provided new insights into the role of inflammation in COPD. In addition, examination of spontaneous or induced sputum has provided a non-invasive method to investigate inflammatory cells in the airways of patients with COPD. Studies have reported increased numbers of neutrophils in the intraluminal space in stable COPD. Bronchial biopsy studies have described inflammation in the bronchi in patients with chronic bronchitis with and without airway obstruction, and shown that activated T-lymphocytes are prominent in the proximal airways. Macrophages are also a prominent feature and, in contrast to asthma, in chronic bronchitis the CD8 suppressor T-lymphocyte subset predominates rather than the CD4 helper subset. Neutrophils are present, particularly in the glands, and become more prominent as the disease progresses. Bronchial biopsies taken from patients during mild exacerbations of chronic bronchitis indicate increased numbers of eosinophils in the bronchial wall, although far fewer than are present in exacerbations of asthma; increased numbers of neutrophils are also observed. Unlike those in patients with asthma, these cells do not appear to have degranulated. Eosinophils may not be prominent in severe exacerbations.

Several studies using bronchoalveolar lavage or, more recently, using spontaneous or induced sputum, have demonstrated intraluminal inflammation in the airspaces of patients with chronic bronchitis with or without airway obstruction. In stable chronic bronchitis, the high percentage of intraluminal neutrophils is associated with the presence of neutrophil chemotactic factors, including interleukin-8 (IL-8) and leukotriene B4, and other inflammatory mediators. There is also evidence that the airspace inflammation in patients with chronic bronchitis persists following smoking cessation if the production of sputum persists, although cough and sputum improve in most smokers who quit. Some preliminary studies suggest that the inflammatory changes present in the large airways may reflect those present in the small airways and perhaps in the alveolar walls.

Chronic inflammation of the bronchial wall is also associated with connective tissue changes that include increased amounts of smooth muscle and degenerative changes in the airway cartilages as well as increased vascularity.

Small-airways disease/bronchiolitis

The smaller bronchi and bronchioles < 2 mm in diameter are a major site of airway obstruction in COPD. Inflammation in the small airways is among the earliest changes to be found in asymptomatic cigarette smokers, and considerable changes in these airways can occur without giving rise to symptoms or alteration in spirometry measurements. Hence, this region in the lung is often referred to as the 'silent zone'. The pattern of inflammatory cell changes in the small airways resembles that in the larger airways, including the predominance of CD8+ lymphocytes and the increase in the CD8:CD4 ratio.

The mechanisms leading to the increase in peripheral airway resistance include several distinct processes: destruction of the alveolar support, loss of elastic recoil in the parenchyma that provides this support, and structural narrowing of the airway lumen. The lumen may be occluded by mucus and cells. Mucosal ulceration, goblet cell hyperplasia and squamous cell metaplasia may be present in addition to fibrosis and mesenchymal cell accumulation. As the condition progresses, structural remodeling may occur, characterized by increased collagen content and scar tissue formation that narrows the airways and produces fixed airway obstruction (Figure 1.2).

Pulmonary emphysema

Pulmonary emphysema is defined in structural and pathological terms as abnormal permanent enlargement of airspaces distal to the terminal bronchioles accompanied by destruction of their walls. The terms used to describe emphysema are based on the anatomy of the normal lung, where a secondary lobule is defined as that part of the lung that contains several terminal bronchioles surrounded by connective tissue septa. An acinus is that part of the lung parenchyma supplied by a

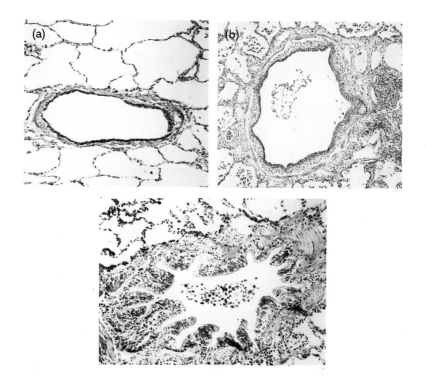

Figure 1.2 Histological sections of peripheral airways. (a) Section from a cigarette smoker with normal lung function, showing a nearly normal airway. (b) Section from a patient with small-airways disease, showing inflammatory exudate in the wall and lumen of the airway. (c) A more advanced case of small-airways disease, with reduced lumen, structural reorganization of the airway wall, increased smooth muscle and deposition of peribronchiolar connective tissue. Images reproduced with the kind permission of Professor James C Hogg, University of British Columbia.

single terminal bronchiole. Therefore, each secondary lobule contains several terminal bronchioles and thus several acini.

Emphysema is classified by the pattern of the enlarged airspaces on the cut surface of the fixed inflated lung (Figure 1.3). Airspace enlargement can be identified macroscopically when the airspace size reaches 1 mm. Absence of obvious fibrosis is a prerequisite in most definitions of emphysema; histologically, however, fibrosis has been recognized in the region of the terminal or respiratory bronchioles as

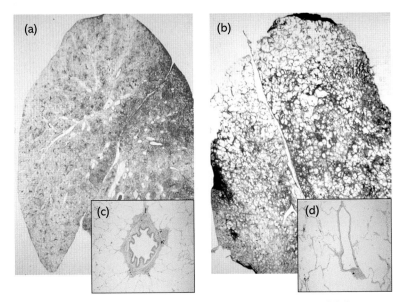

Figure 1.3 (a) Paper-mounted whole lung section of normal lung. (b) Paper-mounted whole lung section from a lung with severe centrilobular emphysema (note that the centrilobular form is more extensive in the upper regions of the lung). (c) Histological section of normal small airway and surrounding alveoli connecting with attached alveolar walls. (d) Histological section showing emphysema, with enlarged alveolar spaces, loss of alveolar wall and attachments and collapsed airways.

part of a respiratory bronchiolitis which occurs in smokers, and lung collagen content is increased in mild emphysema. Three principal types of emphysema are recognized according to the distribution of the enlarged airspaces within the acinar unit (Figure 1.4): centriacinar, panacinar and periacinar (paraseptal) emphysema, the last being the least common. Other, less frequent forms are also discussed briefly here.

Centriacinar and panacinar emphysema can occur alone or in combination. There is still debate over whether the two types represent different disease processes and hence have different etiologies, or whether panacinar emphysema is a progression from centriacinar emphysema. The association with cigarette smoking is certainly clearer for centriacinar than panacinar emphysema, although smokers can develop both types. Those with centriacinar emphysema appear to

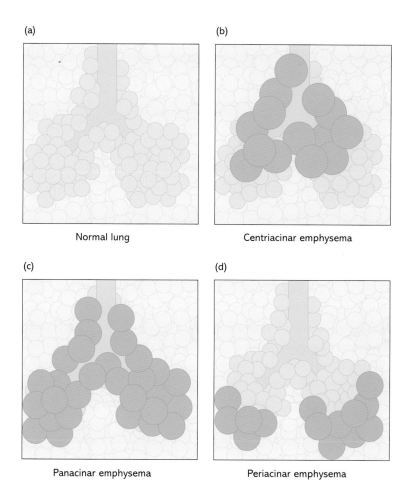

(a)

Normal lung

(b)

Centriacinar emphysema

(c)

Panacinar emphysema

(d)

Periacinar emphysema

Figure 1.4 A diagrammatic representation of the distribution of the abnormal airspaces within the acinar unit in the three major types of emphysema. (a) Acinar unit in a normal lung (although the illustration shows a clearly defined area for the purposes of clarity, it must be remembered that adjacent acinar units intercommunicate and are not necessarily demarcated by septa). (b) Centriacinar emphysema: focal enlargement of the airspaces around the respiratory bronchiole. (c) Panacinar (panlobular) emphysema: confluent, even involvement of the acinar unit. (d) Periacinar (paraseptal or distal acinar) emphysema: peripherally distributed enlarged airspaces where the acinar unit butts against a fixed structure such as the pleura.

have more abnormalities in their small airways than those with predominantly panacinar emphysema.

Centriacinar (centrilobular) emphysema is characterized by initial clustering of the enlarged airspaces around the terminal bronchiole. It is more prominent in the upper zones of the upper and lower lobes.

Panacinar (panlobular) emphysema has the enlarged airspaces distributed throughout the acinar unit. The destruction of the acinus is more uniform, and all of the acini within the secondary lobule are involved. In contrast to centriacinar emphysema, panacinar emphysema appears to be more severe in the lower lobe, but can be found anywhere in the lungs. It is associated with α_1-proteinase inhibitor deficiency, but it can also be found in cases where no clear-cut genetic abnormality has been identified.

Periacinar (paraseptal or distal acinar) emphysema is characterized by enlargement of the airspaces along the edge of the acinar unit, but only where it abuts against a fixed structure such as the pleura or a vessel. Periacinar emphysema is usually of little clinical significance unless it occurs extensively in a subpleural position, when it may be associated with pneumothorax.

Unilateral emphysema or McLeod syndrome occurs as a complication of the severe childhood infections rubella or adenovirus.

Congenital lobular emphysema is a developmental abnormality affecting newborn children.

Scar or irregular emphysema comprises enlarged airspaces around the margins of a scar unrelated to the structure of the acinus.

Bullae are localized areas of emphysema that have overdistended. Conventionally, only lesions over 1 cm in size are described as bullae. Bullae arise in areas of lung which have been locally destroyed, although this destruction does not have to be a result of emphysema; it can also occur from lytic or traumatic causes. They have been described in patients with tuberculosis, sarcoidosis, AIDS and trauma. The origins of bullae remain obscure. In the minority of cases, around 20%, the surrounding lung is normal, but most bullae are associated with more generalized emphysema and chronic airway obstruction. Bullae have been classified according to their size and position.

- Type I bullae have a narrow neck, attached to a mushroom-like expansion into the pleural space.
- Type II bullae have a broader neck and spring from distension of a moderate area of emphysema.
- Type III bullae occur in an area of severe emphysema within the lung and have no pleural reflection.

Grading of emphysema. The severity of emphysema can be measured either macroscopically or microscopically in resected lung specimens. Macroscopic emphysema can be assessed by the point-counting technique, in which a grid of points is placed over the lung and the numbers of points overlying normal and emphysematous lung are recorded, producing a quantitative assessment of the amount of lung involved. Various emphysema grading techniques have been described; the best known is that which uses a series of paper-mounted cross-sections of lungs with varying degrees of emphysema ranked from 0, for normal lung, to 100, for the most extensive emphysema encountered.

These techniques fail to identify airspaces < 1 mm in diameter and therefore do not measure microscopic emphysema. Microscopic emphysema has been measured using the mean linear intercept, which estimates the diameter of the airspaces, or in terms of the surface area of the alveolus or airspace wall per unit lung volume.

Pulmonary vasculature

The development of chronic alveolar hypoxia in patients with COPD produces characteristic remodeling of the pulmonary arteries. However, other changes occur earlier in the natural history of the disease; the first is thickening of the intima, followed by increase in smooth muscle and infiltration of the vessel wall with inflammatory cells. As the disease progresses, the amounts of smooth muscle, proteoglycans and collagen present in the vessel wall increase and cause it to thicken. Right ventricular hypertrophy and pulmonary hypertension are commonly found in patients with COPD who have chronic hypoxemia. Right ventricular hypertrophy can be measured at postmortem as the Fulton index, which is the ratio of the weight of the left ventricle and the aventricular septum to that of the free right ventricular wall. This ratio is normally greater than 2.2.

Physiological significance

The pathological changes in patients with COPD are complex and may occur to varying extents in the large and small airways and in the alveolar compartment. It is difficult to determine clinically or by respiratory function tests the relative contributions made to airway

---

Key points – pathology

- COPD results from pathological changes in large and small airways (bronchiolitis) and in the alveolar space (emphysema).
- Chronic bronchitis is defined clinically as the production of sputum on most days for at least 3 months a year over at least 2 consecutive years.

- Inflammation occurs in large and small airways and in the alveolar space, involving a number of cells including neutrophils, macrophages and T-lymphocytes, particularly CD8+ lymphocytes.
- Small-airways disease or bronchiolitis can result in inflammation and eventually scarring of the small airways; this is an important pathological change in COPD, which is difficult to assess by respiratory function tests, but may be a major source of airway obstruction.
- Centriacinar emphysema is the commonest variety of emphysema, occurring particularly in smokers, and distributed mainly in the upper lung zones. Panacinar emphysema has a more diffuse distribution with a lower lung zone predominance, and is associated with α_1-antitrypsin deficiency but can also occur in some smokers.
- Bullae are emphysematous spaces > 1 cm in diameter.
- Combinations of these pathological changes occur to varying extents in different individuals with COPD and contribute to the airflow limitation.

obstruction by the different pathological changes. In general, it is thought the smaller bronchi and bronchioles < 2 mm in diameter are the major site of airway obstruction in COPD.

Narrowing of small airways can result from the formation of peribronchiolar scars and consequent contraction. Consistent with this, decreased airway circumference correlates well with airflow limitation in patients with moderately severe COPD when assessed on specimens removed surgically. Emphysema leads to decreased expiratory airflow by different mechanisms. Loss of elastic recoil of the lungs decreases the driving pressure that empties the alveoli and reduces the intraluminal pressure within the terminal airways. Because of this and because of destruction of alveolar attachments that tether the small airways in an open position, small airways can collapse during forced exhalation, resulting in effort-independent limitation of expiratory airflow. Hyperinflation of the lungs with overdistension of alveoli may also lead to airway compression. Symptoms and physiological abnormalities in a given individual may be due to different combinations of lesions at different stages.

Key references

Global Initiative for Chronic Obstructive Lung Disease. Pathogenesis, pathology, and pathophysiology. In: *Global Strategy for the Diagnosis, Management, and Prevention of Chronic Obstructive Pulmonary Disease. NHLBI/WHO Workshop Report*. National Heart, Lung, and Blood Institute (USA), World Health Organization: 2001, updated 2003. www.goldcopd.com.

Lamb D. Pathology. In: Calverley P, Pride N, eds. *Chronic Obstructive Pulmonary Disease*. London: Chapman & Hall, 1996:9–35.

MacNee W. Chronic bronchitis and emphysema. In: Seaton A, Seaton D, Leitch AG, eds. *Crofton and Douglas's Respiratory Diseases 1*. Oxford: Blackwell Science, 2000:616–95.

MacNee W, Donaldson K. Pathogenesis of chronic obstructive pulmonary disease. In: Wardlaw AJ, Hamid QA, eds. *Textbook of Respiratory Cell and Molecular Biology*. London: Martin Dunitz, 2002:99–132.

Saetta M, Turato G, Maestrelli P et al. Cellular and structural bases of chronic obstructive pulmonary disease. *Am J Respir Crit Care Med* 2001;163:1304–9.

Turato G, Zuin R, Miniati M et al. Airway inflammation in severe chronic obstructive pulmonary disease: relationship with lung function and radiologic emphysema. *Am J Respir Crit Care Med* 2002;166:105–10.

The measure most commonly used to monitor the natural history of COPD is the forced expiratory volume in 1 second (FEV_1). This parameter can be readily measured by spirometry (see Chapter 4). Most studies of COPD have relied on the FEV_1 as the key measure for the assessment of the etiology, natural history and susceptibility of individual subjects to the development of COPD.

FEV_1 is justly regarded as the single most important objective measure of COPD for both research and clinical purposes. However, several other clinical parameters independently characterize the features of the disease (see Chapter 4).

Etiology

The conducting airways are fully developed by the 16th week of gestation. Alveolar structures develop both pre- and postnatally, increasing in number in early childhood up to about the age of 8 years. Alveolar size continues to increase with lung growth. Maximal lung function is reached in young adulthood and correlates with the attainment of maximal body size. Women achieve maximal lung function earlier than men due to their earlier growth spurt and epiphyseal closures. After achieving a maximum in young adulthood, lung function remains stable for a decade or so and then begins to decline at a slowly increasing rate. On average, FEV_1 declines at about 20 mL/year after the age of 30, and up to 30 mL/year by age 70.

Risk factors

Low maximal attained lung function increases the risk of excessive loss of lung function in later life. Not surprisingly, a variety of early life events can increase the risk for the development of COPD, presumably by affecting lung growth and development. Individuals with low birth weight, for example, have been shown to have both a reduced maximal attained lung function in young adult life and reduced lung function in older age. Some childhood infections have been reported both to reduce lung function in adulthood and to increase the risk of pulmonary symptoms. Interestingly, these infections may affect lung function in several ways. In addition to acutely altering lung growth and development, some infections may have direct effects in later life. Specifically, small portions of some viral genomes can be chronically incorporated and expressed in lung cells. Such expression may predispose individuals to inflammation and lung damage in later life.

Airway hyperreactivity is also a risk factor for the development of COPD. It is measured by challenging individuals with low doses of the acetylcholine analog methacholine or with histamine. The challenge results in constriction of airway smooth muscle and a reduction in airflow, usually measured by FEV_1. In hyperreactive airways, a lower dose of methacholine is required to reduce airflow by 20% (Figure 2.1).

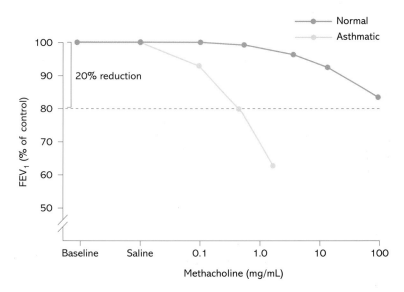

Figure 2.1 Airflow in hyperreactive airways is reduced by a lower dose of methacholine than airflow in normal airways. Here the normal and asthmatic responses to a methacholine challenge are plotted in terms of the FEV_1, expressed as a percentage of the baseline value, against methacholine dose. Adapted with permission from Baum GL, Crapo JD, Celli B, Karlinsky J, eds. *Textbook of Pulmonary Diseases*, 6th edn, vol I. Philadelphia: Lippincott Raven, 1998:209.

Asthma is characterized by increased airway reactivity. The greater risk of developing COPD among individuals with increased reactivity therefore suggests a link between asthma and COPD. Consistent with this, a proportion of asthmatic patients appear to have an accelerated rate of lung function decline, suggesting that they are developing COPD.

Cigarette smoking is the most important etiologic factor for the development of COPD. There is a highly significant dose and duration effect, with smokers having lower lung function the more and longer they smoke. There is, however, considerable individual variation. Some non-smokers, for example, have impaired lung function. Approximately 20% of COPD patients (see below) are lifelong non-smokers. Conversely, some heavy smokers are able to maintain normal lung function (Figure 2.2).

It is likely that smoking contributes to the development of COPD in several distinct ways and at several different periods over the lifespan of the individual (Table 2.1). As noted above, low birth weight is a risk factor for the development of COPD. Infants born to mothers who smoke are at increased risk of low birth weight. Children who take up smoking before achieving maximal stature have reduced lung growth. Thus, cigarette smoking can decrease maximal attained lung function. Smoking in young adulthood is believed to reduce the 'plateau phase', during which lung function remains stable in young adulthood. Finally, smoking accelerates the rate at which lung function declines in adulthood. Thus, smoking has adverse effects on lung function, and the adverse effects are likely to be greater the earlier an individual is exposed.

Exposure to other substances can also contribute to the development of COPD. These include indoor and outdoor pollution. Importantly, passive exposure to cigarette smoke is an important risk and may contribute to the COPD that develops in non-smokers. Individuals exposed to dusts and fumes who also smoke cigarettes have the highest risk.

The mechanisms by which cigarette smoke leads to COPD are under intensive study, as they offer potential opportunities for therapeutic intervention. Smoke is capable of inducing an inflammatory response through a number of mechanisms. It induces release of proinflammatory

23

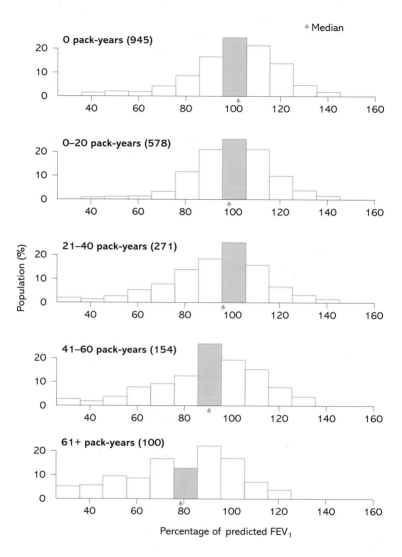

Figure 2.2 Distribution of FEV$_1$ values as a percentage of predicted value for groups with differing smoking histories. Data from Burrows et al. 1979.

mediators from epithelial cells present in the lower respiratory tract, as well as from resident macrophages. It can also activate complement. Hence, the inflammation that is characteristically present in the lungs of smokers probably results from activation of multiple pathways. The

TABLE 2.1

Mechanisms by which smoking may contribute to COPD

Prenatal exposure
- Decreased lung development
- Low birth weight

Childhood
- Decreased lung growth

Adulthood
- Accelerated onset of lung function decline
- Lung destruction
- Impaired lung repair

mediators released by inflammatory cells and parenchymal cells recruited and stimulated by cigarette smoke are capable of inducing lung damage. These mediators include reactive oxygen species, active proteinases and toxic peptides. In addition, cigarette smoke can decrease levels of antioxidants and antiproteinases that serve to mitigate damage caused by these toxic moieties. These effects therefore tip the balance in the lung toward tissue damage both by increasing the production of toxic mediators and by decreasing defenses.

Smoke may also alter the ability of the lung to repair itself. This feature may resemble the widely recognized adverse effect smoke has on wound healing systemically. In other words, smoke can both increase tissue damage and impair the ability to repair that damage.

The complex interactions between cigarette smoke and the lungs of smokers suggest multiple steps at which individual susceptibility may vary. Consistent with this, smokers show considerable heterogeneity in their susceptibility to developing COPD. Importantly, there appear to be strong genetic components. Both smoking and non-smoking siblings of individuals with established COPD are at greatly increased risk for lower lung function than are siblings of individuals without COPD. It is likely that a number of specific genetic alterations will affect susceptibility to COPD.

Genetic factors. Several candidate genes have been suggested
(Table 2.2). To date, the only widely accepted genetic association with
COPD is α_1-proteinase inhibitor deficiency (α_1-antitrypsin deficiency).
People deficient in α_1-proteinase inhibitor are at increased risk for
developing COPD even if they do not smoke. If such individuals smoke,
they are likely to develop severe COPD at a particularly early age
(Figure 2.3). α_1-proteinase inhibitor is a major inhibitor of serine
proteinases, including neutrophil elastase; thus it is postulated that
deficiency in α_1-proteinase inhibitor results in excess activity of
neutrophil elastase and therefore tissue destruction and emphysema.
However, only some non-smokers with α_1-proteinase inhibitor
deficiency develop emphysema. Some maintain normal lung function
throughout life. This indicates the importance of other factors.

TABLE 2.2

Genetic factors possibly related to COPD risk

- α_1-proteinase inhibitor
- α_1-antichymotrypsin
- α_2-macroglobulin
- Matrix metalloproteinase-1
- Matrix metalloproteinase-12
- Microsomal epoxide hydrolase
- Glutathione S transferase
- Heme oxygenase 1
- Cytochrome P450 1A1
- Vitamin D binding protein
- Tumor necrosis factor α
- Interleukin-1
- Interleukin-1 receptor antagonist
- Cystic fibrosis transmembrane regulator
- α_2-adrenergic receptor
- ABO-secretor status
- Microsatellite instability

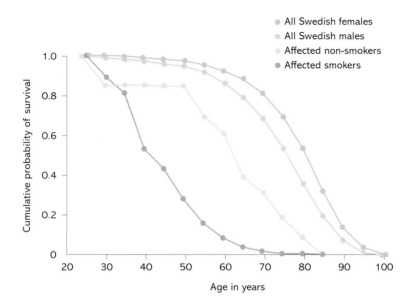

Figure 2.3 Cumulative probability of survival after age 20 for smoking and non-smoking individuals with α_1-proteinase inhibitor deficiency compared with the total population. Data from Larsson 1978.

Though not yet established, there are hypotheses proposing that several other genes contribute to the development of COPD. Interestingly, many of these candidate genes can affect proteinase or oxidant balance, suggesting mechanisms of action analogous to that of α_1-proteinase inhibitor deficiency.

Inhibition of tissue repair may contribute to the development of COPD alongside the mechanisms that augment tissue destruction. Starvation, for example, has been reported to cause COPD both in humans and in animals. Moreover, starvation can exacerbate proteinase-induced emphysema in animal models. Such a mechanism may have clinical relevance. Many individuals with seemingly stable COPD often deteriorate when their course is complicated by a severe and prolonged intercurrent illness. Among the benefits of careful attention to nutritional balance in such patients might be mitigation of the acceleration of COPD.

Other factors can also contribute. For example, emphysema has been reported in patients with HIV infection. In this context, the inflammation associated with HIV may be a contributing factor independent of cigarette smoke.

Progression of clinical symptoms

Current understanding of the natural history of COPD depends on assessment of FEV_1. Nevertheless, other clinical disease parameters are important, independent of FEV_1. Weight loss, for example, is a bad prognostic sign, with survival in COPD patients being negatively correlated with body mass index (Figure 2.4). Similarly, measures of

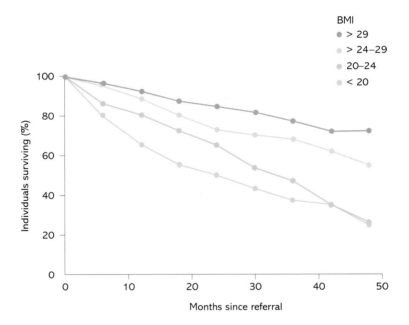

Figure 2.4 Weight as a prognostic sign in COPD: survival is negatively correlated with body mass index. The data represent 400 consecutive COPD patients referred for rehabilitation, who received no special dietary intervention. BMI, body mass index (mass [kg]/height^2 [m^2]). Data from Schols AM, Slangen J, Volovics L, Wouters EF. Weight loss is a reversible factor in the prognosis of chronic obstructive pulmonary disease. *Am J Respir Crit Care Med* 1998;157:1791–7.

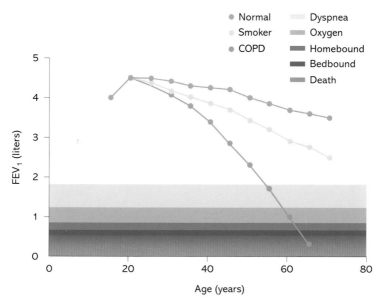

Figure 2.5 The natural history of COPD (adapted from Fletcher 1976 and 1977). The clinical features are related to averages for FEV_1; there are marked individual variations.

health status, sometimes termed 'quality of life', correlate significantly, but weakly, with FEV_1. Other factors such as exacerbations seem to be more important in driving health status, particularly in severely affected individuals.

It is important, therefore, to view the natural history of COPD not only in terms of FEV_1 decline, but also in terms of increasing symptoms. Times of onset of symptoms are depicted in Figure 2.5, but these are averages. Many individual patients will have symptoms at a much earlier stage, and some will progress to very limited airflow without being symptomatic. Some of the variation in symptomatic natural history is probably due to the fact that dyspnea is not directly related to FEV_1. Rather, with exertion, tachypnea ensues. This can lead to dynamic hyperinflation, and it is the increase in inspiratory work that is generally perceived as dyspnea. Many people developing COPD control dyspnea on exertion by decreasing their level of exertion. As a result, they forgo activities as their disease progresses. Often this is

l to aging or is accepted as 'normal' in a smoker, and subjects
ne severely limited before presenting with complaints.

t that subjects with COPD can be compromised at early
stages of the disease without complaining of symptoms is a major
reason for encouraging early diagnosis. Initiation of appropriate
therapy early may improve patient function and quality of life, while
preventing the severe deconditioning that routinely accompanies
progressive COPD. Early recognition and intervention is a major goal
of the new GOLD classification, and contrasts with older staging
systems, in which a greater emphasis was placed on end-stage disease.

Key points – etiology and natural history

- Cigarette smoking is the most important risk factor; about 80%
  of COPD patients are or have been smokers.
- Almost all smokers develop impaired lung function. A diagnosis
  of COPD is made in about 15%, as many do not seek help for
  their functional compromise.
- Other influences, including air pollution and occupational
  exposures, contribute to COPD risk.
- Individual genetic susceptibility probably accounts for the
  heterogeneity of COPD risk.
- It is likely that many specific genetic factors will contribute to
  COPD risk, though only one, α_1-proteinase inhibitor deficiency,
  has been unequivocally identified.
- Asthma may contribute to COPD risk in some individuals.
- Early life events, including compromise of lung development
  and growth, are likely to contribute to the risk of developing
  COPD later.

Key references

Barker DJ, Godfrey KM, Fall C et al. Relation of birth weight and childhood respiratory infection to adult lung function and death from chronic obstructive airways disease. *BMJ* 1991;303:671–5.

Burrows B, Knudson RJ, Cline MG et al. Quantitative relationships between cigarette smoking and ventilatory function. *Am Rev Respir Dis* 1979;115:751–60.

Fletcher C, Peto R, Tinker C, Speizer FE. *The Natural History of Chronic Bronchitis and Emphysema: An Eight-Year Study of Early Chronic Obstructive Lung Disease in Working Men in London.* New York: Oxford University Press, 1976:1–272.

Fletcher C, Peto R. The natural history of chronic airflow obstruction. *BMJ* 1977;1:1645–8.

Larsson C. Natural history and life expectancy in severe α_1-antitrypsin deficiency, Pi Z. *Acta Med Scand* 1978;204:345–51.

O'Donnell DE, Lam M, Webb KA. Measurement of symptoms, lung hyperinflation, and endurance during exercise in chronic obstructive pulmonary disease. *Am J Respir Crit Care Med* 1998;158:1557–65.

Piquette CA, Rennard SI, Snider GL. Chronic bronchitis and emphysema. In: Murray JF, Nadel JA, eds. *Textbook of Respiratory Medicine*, 3rd edn. Philadelphia: WB Saunders, 2000:1187–1245.

Sandford AJ, Joos L, Pare PD. Genetic risk factors for chronic obstructive pulmonary disease. *Curr Opin Pulm Med* 2002;8:87–94.

Schols AM, Mostert R, Soeters PB, Wouters EF. Body composition and exercise performance in patients with chronic obstructive pulmonary disease. *Thorax* 1991;46:695–9.

Clinical features

Symptoms

The characteristic symptom of COPD is breathlessness on exertion, sometimes accompanied by wheeze and cough, which is often, but not invariably, productive. Breathlessness is the symptom which commonly causes the patient to seek medical attention, and it is usually the most disabling of these symptoms. Patients often date the onset of their illness from an episode of worsening cough with sputum production, which leaves them with a degree of chronic breathlessness. However, close questioning will often reveal the presence of a 'smoker's cough' over a period of years, along with the production of small amounts (usually < 60 mL/day) of mucoid sputum, usually predominating in the morning.

Most patients (80%) with COPD will have a smoking history of at least 20 pack-years (1 pack-year is equivalent to smoking 20 cigarettes – 1 pack – per day for 1 year or 10 a day for 2 years) before symptoms develop, commonly in the fifth decade. It is characteristic of patients with COPD to progress through the clinical stages of mild, moderate and severe disease. Symptoms and signs therefore vary in any individual depending on the stage of the disease. Considerable loss of lung function can occur before symptoms become apparent, and many patients may seek medical attention when the disease is in an advanced stage, since COPD is a slowly progressive disorder and patients gradually adapt their lives to their disability. Most smokers expect to cough and be short of breath, so they often dismiss these symptoms of progressive airflow obstruction as a normal consequence of their smoking habit.

Breathlessness is the symptom which causes most disability and is associated with loss of lung function over time. In good health, the body meets the increased oxygen demand produced by exercise by using some of the inspiratory reserve volume of the lungs to increase tidal volume (Figure 3.1). In COPD, because the caliber of the airways

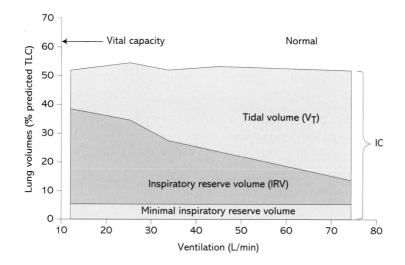

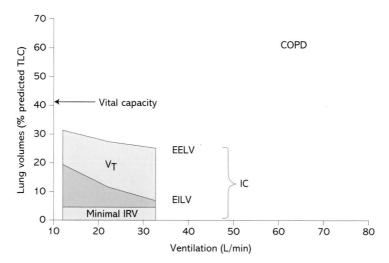

Figure 3.1 In good health, the body meets the increased oxygen demand produced by exercise by using some of the inspiratory reserve volume of the lungs to increase tidal volume. The vertical axes here are presented inverted from the pulmonological convention for clarity. Data from O'Donnell DE, Revill SM, Webb KA. Dynamic hyperinflation and exercise intolerance in chronic obstructive pulmonary disease. *Am J Resp Crit Care Med* 2001;164:770–7. EELV, end expiratory lung volume; EILV, end inspiratory lung volume; IC, inspiratory capacity; IRV, inspiratory reserve volume; TLC, total lung capacity.

is relatively fixed, the inspiratory reserve volume cannot be fully utilized. Overinflation of the lungs with air trapping in the alveoli, particularly when the respiratory rate is increased, leads to increased residual volume at the expense of the inspiratory reserve volume, which worsens breathlessness. Airway collapse due to loss of alveolar support and emphysema causes more air trapping, further increasing the residual volume and increasing breathlessness on exertion. Flattening of the diaphragm when the lungs are overinflated means that the accessory muscles of respiration become increasingly important. The loss of alveolar/capillary surface in COPD, particularly in emphysema, means that the increased demand for oxygen imposed by exercise cannot be met, and this increases the sensation of breathlessness.

In contrast to asthma, where breathlessness is variable, in COPD it is nearly constant, although some patients do report variation, particularly that breathlessness is worse in the morning.

Breathlessness is usually first noted while climbing hills or stairs, carrying heavy loads or hurrying on level ground. The appearance of breathlessness heralds moderate to severe impairment of airway function. By the time the patient seeks medical advice, FEV_1 has usually fallen to around 1–1.5 liters in an average man (30–45% of the expected value). Patients with COPD may adapt their breathing pattern and their behavior to minimize the sensation of breathlessness. Generally, this takes the form of greatly restricted activity.

The perception of breathlessness varies greatly between individuals with the same degree of ventilatory capacity. Breathlessness can be assessed on the modified Borg Scale (Table 3.1), a visual analog scale or the Medical Research Council (MRC) Dyspnea Scale (Table 3.2). Mood is an important determinant of the perception of breathlessness in patients with COPD. When FEV_1 has fallen to 30% or less of the predicted values (equivalent in an average man to an FEV_1 of around 1 liter), breathlessness is usually present on minimal exertion. Severe breathlessness is often affected by changes in temperature and by exposure to dust and fumes. Position has a variable effect on breathlessness. Some patients have severe orthopnea, relieved by leaning forward, whereas others find greatest ease when lying flat.

TABLE 3.1

The modified Borg Scale for assessing breathlessness

Scale	Severity experienced by patient
0	Nothing at all
0.5	Very, very slight (just noticeable)
1	Very slight
2	Slight (light)
3	Moderate
4	Somewhat severe
5	Severe (heavy)
6	
7	Very severe
8	
9	Very, very severe (almost maximal)
10	Maximal

TABLE 3.2

The MRC Dyspnea Scale for assessing breathlessness

Grade	Degree of breathlessness related to activities
0	Not troubled by breathlessness except on strenuous exercise
'1	Short of breath when hurrying or walking up a slight hill
2	Walks slower than contemporaries on the level because of breathlessness, or has to stop for breath when walking at own pace
3	Stops for breath after walking about 100 m or after a few minutes on the level
4	Too breathless to leave the house, or breathless when dressing or undressing
5	Breathless at rest

Cough and sputum production. A productive cough occurs in up to 50% of cigarette smokers. It may either precede or appear simultaneously with the onset of breathlessness, and occurs in association with breathlessness in 75% of patients with COPD. The MRC symptom questionnaire uses cough as a defining symptom of chronic bronchitis, meaning a cough productive of sputum on most days for 3 consecutive months, over 2 consecutive years. Cessation of cigarette smoking produces resolution of the cough in 94% of smokers; however, the airflow limitation often persists. Cough is often worse in the morning, but nocturnal cough does not appear to be increased in stable COPD, in contrast to asthma. In the presence of severe airway obstruction, the generation of high intrathoracic pressures may produce syncope during paroxysms of cough and 'cough fractures' of the ribs. Cough may also be exacerbated by gastroesophageal reflux.

Sputum production is a common, although not a universal, feature of COPD. Sputum is usually white or grey in color and may become mucopurulent green or yellow during exacerbations. However, some patients with COPD have persistently purulent sputum; this may relate to bacterial colonization in the airway. Indeed, it is now recognized that a number of such patients have underlying bronchiectasis. Excessive sputum production (more than 60 mL/day) should raise the possibility of bronchiectasis.

Hemoptysis can occur in exacerbations of COPD in association with infection, but should always be treated seriously; the possibility of underlying bronchial carcinoma should be investigated, since patients with COPD have a high incidence of this condition. The production of copious amounts of frothy sputum, particularly associated with orthopnea, comorbidity of hypertension and/or ischemic heart disease, raises a suspicion of left ventricular failure and pulmonary edema.

Wheeze is a common symptom in COPD but is not universally present and is not specific for the condition. It is not easy to evaluate because of its intermittent nature and the difficulties patients experience in understanding this symptom. Wheeze is due to turbulent airflow through larger airways from various causes including bronchial smooth muscle contraction, structural airway narrowing or the presence of excess airway secretions. Wheeze does not usually wake COPD patients at night as it does asthma patients. The absence of the symptom or signs of wheeze on auscultation of the chest does not exclude a diagnosis of COPD.

Other symptoms. Chest pain is common in patients with COPD, but is often unrelated to the disease itself, and may be due to underlying ischemic heart disease or gastroesophageal reflux. Patients with COPD often complain of chest tightness during exacerbations of breathlessness, particularly during exercise, and sometimes this is difficult to distinguish from ischemic cardiac pain. Pleuritic chest pain may suggest an intercurrent pneumothorax, pneumonia or pulmonary infarction.

Weight loss is a feature of severe COPD and is thought to result from anorexia, decreased calorie intake and increased metabolism.

Psychiatric morbidity, particularly depression, is common in patients with severe COPD, reflecting the social isolation and the chronicity of the disease. Sleep quality is impaired in advanced COPD, which may contribute to the impaired neuropsychiatric performance.

Muscular weakness is a common feature of COPD. It is the best predictor of poor exercise performance, correlating more strongly than either lung function or blood gas measurements. Weakness may be due either to deconditioning or to cellular changes in the skeletal muscle consequent on the inflammatory processes underlying COPD.

Osteoporosis is more common in COPD patients than the general population. This may be due, in part, to concurrent smoking and to the use of glucocorticoids. COPD itself, however, appears to be associated with bone mineral loss.

History

A detailed history is important in COPD. This should include:
- full smoking history
- history of exposure to other risk factors, particularly gases or dusts, and an occupational history
- medical history including asthma, allergy, sinusitis, nasal polyps, respiratory infection in childhood and other respiratory diseases

- family history of COPD or other chronic respiratory disease
- history of symptom development
- history of exacerbations or previous hospitalizations for respiratory disorders
- presence of comorbidity such as heart disease that may also contribute to the restriction of activity
- appropriateness of current medical treatment
- impact of the disease on the patient's life, including limitation of activity, missed work and economic impact, effect on family and feelings of depression or anxiety
- social and family support available to the patient.

COPD is relatively rare among non-smokers and thus details of the patient's exposure to cigarettes, measured in pack-years, is important. Usually, symptomatic COPD develops after 20 pack-years of smoking. Most patients with COPD are over the age of 40. Similar signs in younger patients with much briefer smoking histories should raise suspicion of another condition and lead to a review of the other possible diagnoses or increased genetic susceptibility to COPD such as α_1-antitrypsin deficiency. There is, in general, a dose response relating the number of cigarettes smoked and FEV_1; however, there are huge individual variations, reflecting the varying susceptibility to cigarette smoke. Occupational exposure to dusts has an additive effect on the decline in lung function, as has been shown in coal miners, in whom both smoking and years of dust exposure contribute to the decline in FEV_1. However, the contribution of smoking is three times as great as that of dust exposure in miners.

Physical signs

The physical signs in patients with COPD are not specific to the disease. They depend on the degree of airflow limitation and pulmonary overinflation, and may be virtually absent in patients with mild to moderate disease, so their sensitivity in detecting or excluding COPD is poor. Physical signs of airflow limitation are rarely present until significant impairment of lung function has occurred. Detection of early COPD is possibly only by spirometry or by imaging techniques such as high-resolution computed tomography (HRCT) to assess emphysema.

Breathing pattern in patients with COPD is often characteristic, with a prolonged expiratory phase. Some patients adopt purse-lipped breathing on expiration, which may reduce expiratory airway collapse. The use of the accessory muscles of respiration, particularly the sternomastoids, is often seen in advanced disease; these patients often lean forward, supporting themselves with their arms to fix the shoulder girdle, thus allowing the use of the pectorals and the latissimus dorsi to increase chest wall movement.

Signs of overinflation may be present:

- increased anterior/posterior diameter of the chest ('barrel-shaped chest')
- horizontal ribs, prominence of the sternal angle and wide subcostal angle
- reduced distance between suprasternal notch and cricoid cartilage (normally three fingerbreadths)
- inspiratory tracheal tug.

The horizontal position of the diaphragm acts to pull in the lower ribs during inspiration – Hoover's sign. Increased intrathoracic pressure swings may result in indrawing of the suprasternal and supraclavicular fossae and of the intercostal muscles. Percussion of the chest may show decreased hepatic and cardiac dullness, indicating overinflation. A useful sign of gross overinflation is the absence of a dull percussion note, normally due to the underlying heart, over the lower end of the sternum.

Breath sounds may have a prolonged expiratory phase, or may be uniformly diminished, particularly in the advanced stages of the disease. Wheeze may be heard by the unaided ear, at the patient's mouth if necessary, and may be variably present on auscultation both on inspiration and expiration. Crackles may be present, particularly at the lung bases, but are usually scanty, vary with coughing and cannot be distinguished from the coarse crackles of bronchiectasis or fine respiratory crackles of fibrosis or left ventricular failure.

Different degrees of tachypnea may be present in patients with severe COPD, and prolonged forced expiratory time (> 5 seconds) can be a useful indicator of airway obstruction.

Physical appearance may also yield a number of signs. Tar-stained fingers are an indication of the smoking habit. In advanced disease, cyanosis may be present, indicating hypoxemia, but may be influenced by the background lighting or accentuated by polycythemia, and therefore this sign is fairly subjective. The flapping tremor associated with hypercapnia is neither sensitive nor specific, and the often reported papilledema associated with severe hypercapnia is in fact rarely seen.

Weight loss may also be apparent in advanced disease, as well as a reduction in muscle mass. Finger clubbing is not a manifestation of COPD and should suggest the possibility of complicating bronchial neoplasm, bronchiectasis or lung fibrosis.

Cardiovascular signs. Overinflation of the chest produces difficulty in localizing the apex beat and reduces the cardiac dullness. The characteristic signs that indicate the presence or consequences of pulmonary arterial hypertension may be difficult to detect in advanced cases. The heave of right ventricular hypertrophy may be palpable at the lower left sternal edge or in the subcostal angle. Heart sounds are generally soft, although the second heart sound may be exaggerated in the second left intercostal space in the presence of pulmonary hypertension. Splitting of the second heart sound with an increased pulmonic component may be present. There may be a right-sided gallop rhythm, with a third sound audible in the fourth intercostal space to the left of the sternum, or in the epigastrium. The jugular venous pressure can be difficult to estimate in patients with COPD as it varies widely with respiration and is difficult to discern because of the prominent accessory muscle activity. When the fluid retention of cor pulmonale occurs, there may be evidence of functional tricuspid incompetence, producing a pansystolic murmur at the left sternal edge.

Peripheral vasodilation accompanies hypercapnia, producing warm peripheries with a high-volume pulse. Pitting peripheral edema may be present as a result of fluid retention. However, other causes of edema, such as venous stasis, low serum albumin and deep venous thrombosis, should be considered.

The liver may be tender and pulsatile, and a prominent 'v' wave may be visible in the jugular venous pulse. The liver may also be palpable below the right costal margin as a result of the low diaphragm due to the overinflation of the lungs.

Types of clinical presentation

Many smokers accept the development of exertional dyspnea and cough with sputum production as an inevitable consequence of the smoking habit, and therefore often present to their doctor when the disease is at a fairly advanced stage. Relatively few patients are picked up early in the disease process thanks to a physician with a high index of suspicion or as a result of screening by spirometry. Repeated spirometry over the course of several years will identify smokers with a rapid decline in FEV_1, who could be targeted for smoking cessation and early therapeutic intervention.

Some patients present initially to hospital or to their GP during an exacerbation of the disease and claim that they had no significant symptoms until that time. However, close questioning often reveals the presence of progressive symptoms.

Two clinical patterns have been described, which are now recognized to be at either end of a clinical spectrum – the so-called 'pink puffers' and 'blue bloaters'. The pink and puffing patient is thin and breathless and preserves blood gas values until late in the course of the disease, and therefore does not develop pulmonary hypertension until the disease is very advanced. By contrast, the blue and bloated patient develops hypoxemia and hypercapnia earlier, and thus also the complications of edema and secondary polycythemia. Most patients lie between these two extremes. These 'phenotypes' are not indicative of emphysema or bronchitis, as was once thought, but clearly indicate the varied systemic manifestations of COPD.

Systemic effects of COPD

Traditionally, COPD is regarded as a disease of the lungs characterized by progressive symptoms and decline of lung function. Therapeutic strategies such as bronchodilators and steroids have therefore been used for relieving symptoms in association with improving airflow limitation.

Exercise limitation is a frequent complaint in COPD and is usually explained on the basis of the increased work of breathing caused by airflow limitation. However, almost half the patients with COPD stop exercising because of leg fatigue, not because of breathlessness. This suggests that skeletal muscle dysfunction is an important factor in the symptom complex. Skeletal muscle in patients with COPD is abnormal, and this is not entirely due to their sedentary lifestyle. The mechanisms of the abnormal skeletal muscle function in COPD are not yet fully understood, although some may be due to limited oxygen delivery.

Many COPD patients lose weight during the course of their disease. This phenomenon is of prognostic value, independent of the more traditional prognostic factors related to FEV_1 and PaO_2 (the partial pressure of oxygen in arterial blood). The mechanisms underlying the weight loss are unclear, but may relate to increased metabolic rate, tissue hypoxia and systemic inflammation.

COPD is characterized by an excessive inflammatory process in the lung parenchyma in response to inhaled particles or gases. Evidence of inflammation has also been detected in the systemic circulation, such as markers of oxidative stress, elevated levels of cytokines and activation of circulating leukocytes.

Spectrum of disease

Many national and international guidelines for COPD have used a simple classification of disease severity based on spirometry. The most recent classification from the Global Initiative for Chronic Obstructive Lung Disease also includes symptoms (see Table 4.1, page 47).

Key points – clinical features

- COPD is uncommon, but not unknown, in those who do not smoke.
- Usually there is a significant smoking history of at least 20 pack-years. For those with lesser smoking histories or for younger individuals, consider an alternative diagnosis or genetic predisposition such as α_1-antitrypsin deficiency.
- The commonest and most distressing symptom in COPD is breathlessness on exertion.
- Symptoms and signs often only present at an advanced stage of the disease.
- Clinical signs may not be apparent in mild disease. They include signs of overinflation, prominent use of accessory muscles of respiration, weight loss, expiratory wheeze, cyanosis, peripheral edema and raised jugular venous pressure.

Key references

Calverley PMA, Geogopoulos D. Chronic obstructive pulmonary disease: symptoms and signs. In: Postma DS, Siafakis NM, eds. *Management of Chronic Obstructive Pulmonary Disease. Eur Respir Monogr* 1998;3:6–24.

MacNee W. Chronic bronchitis and emphysema. In: Seaton A, Seaton D, Leitch AG, eds. *Crofton and Douglas's Respiratory Diseases 1.* Oxford: Blackwell Science, 2000:616–95.

Spirometry

The most important disturbance of respiratory function in COPD is obstruction to forced expiratory flow. The degree of airflow obstruction cannot be predicted from the symptoms and signs, and therefore assessment of the degree and the progression of airway obstruction should be encouraged in both primary and secondary care. To identify patients early in the course of the disease, spirometry should be performed for those who have chronic cough and sputum production and for those at risk, such as smokers, even if they have no dyspnea. In the early stages of the disease, conventional spirometry may reveal no abnormality. This is because the earliest changes in COPD affect the alveolar walls and small airways. The resulting modest increase in peripheral airway resistance is not reflected in the conventional spirometric measurements. A reduction in forced expiratory volume relative to vital capacity may, however, be a more sensitive measure. Similarly, sequential measures, which track changes in lung function, may also be more sensitive indicators. Spirometry is the most robust test of airflow limitation in patients with COPD.

Spirometry assesses the volume of exhaled air over time and is performed with the patient exhaling from a maximum inhalation to a maximum exhalation using maximum force to blow out all the air as hard and as fast as possible. In healthy individuals this forced expiratory maneuver can be completed in 3–4 seconds, but in patients with increasing airflow limitation it may take up to 15 seconds. The volume of air exhaled is plotted on a graph against the time taken to reach the maximum exhalation (Figure 4.1). Three indices can then be derived:

- FEV_1 – forced expiratory volume in 1 second
- FVC – forced vital capacity, the total volume of the air that can be exhaled from a maximum inhalation to a maximum exhalation
- FEV_1:FVC – the ratio of FEV_1 to FVC, expressed as a percentage.

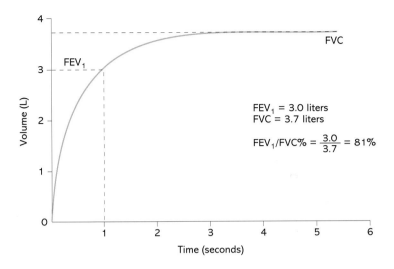

Figure 4.1 Normal spirometry (volume–time trace).

FEV$_1$ and FVC are expressed in absolute values in liters and also as a percentage of the predicted values for the individual depending on their age, height, gender and ethnic origin. Values within ± 20% of the predicted values are considered to be within the normal range. Thus an FEV$_1$ over 80% of the predicted value is considered to be normal. Under normal circumstances 70–80% of the total volume of the air in the lungs (FVC) should be exhaled in the first second. In other words, normally the FEV$_1$:FVC ratio is 70–80%. When airflow through the airways is obstructed, it is not possible to exhale so much air in the first second, and the FEV$_1$:FVC ratio falls. Levels below 70% indicate airflow obstruction (Figure 4.2). An FEV$_1$:FVC ratio below the normal range is a diagnostic criterion for COPD. The GOLD guidelines further stage COPD severity based on the FEV$_1$ as a percentage of the predicted value (Table 4.1).

It is important that a volume plateau is reached in spirometry. This can take 15 seconds or more in a patient with severe airway obstruction. If this maneuver is not carried out properly, the FVC can be underestimated. Many spirometers currently in use substitute FEV$_6$ for FVC. Such instruments therefore underestimate the vital capacity,

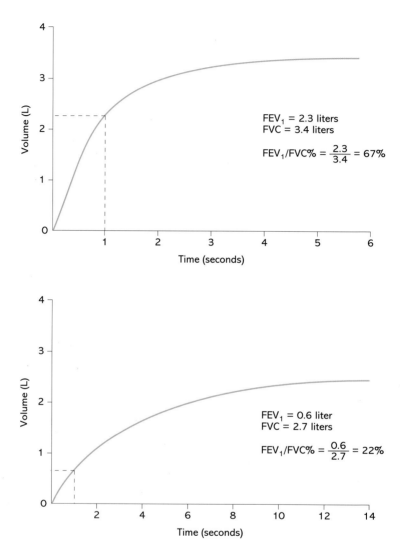

Figure 4.2 (a) Spirometry showing mild obstruction. (b) Spirometry showing severe obstruction.

and hence yield artificially elevated FEV_1:FVC ratios. This limitation is not felt to be a major impediment for the diagnosis of COPD (the criterion being a ratio < 70%), but reduces the reliability of the ratio as a gauge of disease severity.

TABLE 4.1

GOLD classification of severity of COPD

Stage	Characteristics
0: At risk	• Normal spirometry
	• Chronic symptoms (cough, sputum production)
I: Mild COPD	• FEV_1:FVC < 70%
	• $FEV_1 \geq 80\%$ predicted
	• With or without chronic symptoms (cough, sputum production)
II: Moderate COPD	• FEV_1:FVC < 70%
	• $50\% \leq FEV_1 < 80\%$ predicted
III: Severe COPD	• FEV_1:FVC < 70%
	• $30\% \leq FEV_1 < 50\%$ predicted
IV: Very severe COPD	• FEV_1:FVC < 70%
	• $FEV_1 < 30\%$ predicted or $FEV_1 < 50\%$ predicted plus respiratory failure or clinical signs of right heart failure

FEV_1, postbronchodilator forced expiratory volume in 1 second; FVC, forced vital capacity
Source: GOLD Workshop Report Executive Summary, April 2003 (www.goldcopd.com)

Since FEV_1 is effort-dependent, traces should be checked to ensure that maximum effort has been achieved and that full expiration has been performed. The FEV_1 is very reproducible and varies by less than 170 mL between maneuvers if the test is carried out correctly. The test reproducibility is an excellent measure of the effort exerted by the patient and the quality of the test. In contrast to maximal efforts, which are highly reproducible, submaximal efforts are highly variable. Therefore, reproducibility of the tests to within ± 2% is generally regarded as a measure of satisfactory test quality. Many modern spirometers can perform such assessments internally. The FVC also depends on effort, particularly during the latter part of the maneuver, and results are more variable. To avoid the effect of airway collapse in patients with COPD during a forced expiratory maneuver, it is suggested that a relaxed, or slow, vital capacity (VC) measurement, in which patients exhale at their own pace after maximum inhalation, should be used. The slow VC is often 0.5 liters greater than the FVC. With increasing airflow obstruction it takes longer to exhale and the early slope of the volume–time trace becomes less steep (Figure 4.2).

In airway obstruction, the FEV_1 is reduced both as a volume and as a percentage of the predicted value. The FVC also falls, but less than the FEV_1, so that the FEV_1:FVC ratio decreases (Figure 4.2). By contrast, in restrictive defects, such as lung fibrosis or chest-wall deformity, the airway size remains normal, but both FEV_1 and FVC are reduced, so the ratio remains above 70% (Figure 4.3).

In assessing FEV_1, the following points should be remembered.
- Patients should be clinically stable, i.e. at least 4 weeks must have passed since the last exacerbation.
- If patients have taken a bronchodilator, results may be improved from 'baseline'.
- Patients should be sitting in an upright position.
- An adequate explanation of the technique should be given.
- Patients should be asked to take a maximum breath in and then place their lips around the mouthpiece, forming an airtight seal.

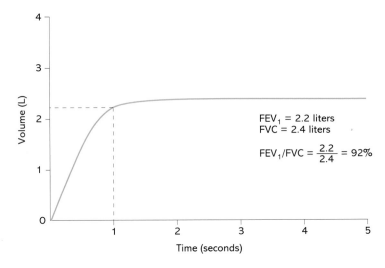

$FEV_1 = 2.2$ liters
$FVC = 2.4$ liters

$$FEV_1/FVC = \frac{2.2}{2.4} = 92\%$$

Figure 4.3 Spirometry of a restrictive defect; the ratio FEV_1:FVC is within the normal range.

- Patients should then be encouraged to exhale as hard, as fast and as completely as possible.
- Adequate time should be allowed for recovery between exhalations, with a maximum of six forced maneuvers being performed in one session.
- Three technically satisfactory maneuvers giving similar results should be carried out.
- At least two readings of FEV_1 should be within 100 mL or 5% of each other.

Patients with COPD typically show a decrease in both FEV_1 and FEV_1:FVC ratio (the latter being a more sensitive measure of early airflow limitation). The degree of spirometric abnormality generally reflects the severity of COPD.

Peak expiratory flow

Peak expiratory flow (PEF) can either be read directly from the flow–volume loop (see below) or measured with a handheld peak flow meter. It is a simple, quick and inexpensive way of measuring airflow obstruction, and has been particularly useful for repeated measurements in asthmatic patients to reveal spontaneous diurnal variation or variations in response to therapy. The PEF meter measures the maximal flow rate that can be maintained over 10 ms; it is most effective for monitoring changes in airflow in an individual over time and has less value in diagnosis. In COPD there is little daily change in PEF and many of the variations are often within the error of the measurement. Although repeated measurements of PEF can be used in place of FEV_1, single measurements are not useful as the variation is so high. There are several theoretical reasons why FEV_1 is a better test than PEF in the diagnosis and assessment of COPD (see Table 4.2).

Reversibility testing

Bronchodilators. The main objectives of a bronchodilator reversibility test in COPD are:
- to help distinguish those patients with marked reversibility who have underlying asthma

TABLE 4.2

Reasons why FEV$_1$ is the measurement of choice in COPD

- It is a reproducible and objective measurement. There are well-defined normal ranges that allow for the effects of age, race and sex

- It is relatively simple and quick to measure and can be measured at all stages of disease

- The forced expiratory maneuver records not only FEV$_1$ but also FVC. An FEV$_1$:FVC ratio < 70% is diagnostic of airway obstruction. If the ratio is normal (> 70%) and the test was performed well, the pattern is not obstructive and the diagnosis is not COPD

- PEF measurements cannot determine whether values are low because of obstruction or restriction

- The variance of repeated FEV$_1$ measurements in the same person is well documented and is low

- Studies of mortality and disability have shown that the FEV$_1$ predicts future mortality from COPD and from other respiratory and cardiac diseases

- Serial measurements provide evidence of disease progression

- In COPD the relationship between PEF and FEV$_1$ is poor

- PEF may underestimate the degree of airway obstruction in COPD

- FEV$_1$ is better related to prognosis and disability than FEV$_1$:FVC because the FVC depends on effort and is therefore more variable

FEV$_1$, forced expiratory volume in 1 s; FVC, forced vital capacity; PEF, peak expiratory flow

- to establish the post-bronchodilator FEV$_1$, which is the best predictor of long-term prognosis
- to establish the best obtainable lung function.

There is no agreement on a standardized method of assessing reversibility. Usually changes in the FEV$_1$ or PEF are monitored, but reversibility could also be determined as a change in static lung volumes after administration of a bronchodilator.

The use of bronchodilator testing in patients with COPD is limited by the variability of the FEV$_1$ measurement itself, and by the fact that by definition patients with COPD may have only a small degree of reversibility, which is often within the error of the measurement.

Bronchodilator reversibility tests can also vary from day to day depending on the degree of bronchomotor tone. A change in FEV_1 that exceeds 170 mL can be considered not to have occurred by chance. Most guidelines recommend that changes should be considered significant only if they exceed 200 mL. In addition to this absolute change in FEV_1, a percentage change of 12% over baseline has been suggested as significant by the American Thoracic Society and the GOLD guidelines, whereas an improvement of 15% over baseline FEV_1 and a 200 mL absolute change has been suggested by European Respiratory Society and British Thoracic Society guidelines.

Another approach to measuring reversibility is to express the change in FEV_1 as a percentage of the maximum potential change, which is the predicted value minus the baseline value.

Reversibility testing with a bronchodilator is generally indicated only at the time of diagnosis. Bronchodilator testing should usually be undertaken only in patients with stage II (moderate) COPD and above, and reversibility testing should be conducted during a period of clinical stability, with a high dose of bronchodilator in order not to miss a significant response. The high dose can be delivered by means of a nebulizer. An alternative method is to deliver a smaller dose of the drug by giving repeated doses from a metered-dose inhaler through a large-volume spacer. The usual recommended protocol for testing bronchial reversibility is shown in Table 4.3. Improvement of lung function to normal suggests a diagnosis of asthma without the presence of COPD.

Daily variations in airway smooth muscle tone may affect the response to bronchodilators in patients with COPD. Thus when airway smooth muscle tone is higher and FEV_1 is therefore lower, a response to bronchodilators may be more likely than when muscle tone is lower and FEV_1 higher. One third of those patients who are initially shown to have a response to a bronchodilator may, on retesting on a different day, have no response. Conversely, patients who do not show a significant FEV_1 response to a bronchodilator can still benefit symptomatically from long-term bronchodilator treatment.

> TABLE 4.3
>
> **Guidelines for bronchodilator reversibility testing**
>
> - Withhold all bronchodilators for sufficient time for therapeutic effect to abate
>
> - Record FEV_1 before and 15 minutes after giving salbutamol (albuterol), 2.5–5 mg, or nebulized terbutaline, 5–10 mg
>
> - Record (preferably on a separate occasion) FEV_1 before and 30 minutes after nebulized ipratropium bromide, 500 µg
>
> - Record (on a separate occasion) FEV_1 before and 30 minutes after a combination of salbutamol (albuterol) or terbutaline and ipratropium
>
> Salbutamol is the recommended international non-proprietary name favored by the WHO, albuterol is the official generic name in the USA

Corticosteroids. Reversibility after administration of corticosteroids is observed in 10–20% of patients with clinically stable COPD. Whether all patients with symptomatic COPD should have formal assessment of corticosteroid reversibility remains controversial. Those patients who have previously shown a response to nebulized bronchodilators are more likely to show a response to corticosteroids. However, it is not possible to predict the response to corticosteroids in any individual patient. Corticosteroid reversibility tests are usually performed during a period of clinical stability. Prednisolone, 30 mg/day, is given for 2 weeks and spirometry is recorded before and immediately at the end of the trial. An alternative and potentially safer approach is to give a 6-week/3-month trial of inhaled corticosteroids such as beclomethasone, 1000 µg/day, or equivalent.

The criteria for a positive response are the same as in bronchodilator reversibility testing: 200 mL and 15% improvement in the FEV_1 over baseline. Another criterion is an improvement of 20% or more in the mean PEF over the first 5 days and the last 5 days of a treatment trial. The response to corticosteroids is best evaluated with respect to the postbronchodilator FEV_1; that is, the postbronchodilator FEV_1 is measured, and then the further improvement achieved by glucocorticoid, since postbronchodilator FEV_1 is the most reliable and least variable measurement from day to day. Improvements in symptoms or exercise tolerance following glucocorticoids may occur in those who show no significant FEV_1 response.

Specialized lung function tests

Flow–volume loops. Many spirometers plot expiratory flow rate through the entire expiration at the same time as a standard volume–time trace. The PEF, which is sustained for 10 ms, represents flow only in larger airways. However, the flow–volume trace interprets flow from all generations of the airways and may be more helpful than PEF in detecting early airway narrowing in smaller airways (Figure 4.4). Expiratory flow rates at 75% or 50% of vital capacity have been used as a measure of airflow limitation, and provide complementary information to that obtained from the usual volume–time plot. There are problems with the reproducibility of these measurements, so that values must fall below 50% of the predicted values to be considered abnormal. Flows at lung volumes below 50% of vital capacity were previously considered to be an indicator of small-airways dysfunction, but probably provide no more clinically useful information than measurements of the FEV_1. Examples of flow–volume loops in airflow obstruction are shown in Figure 4.5.

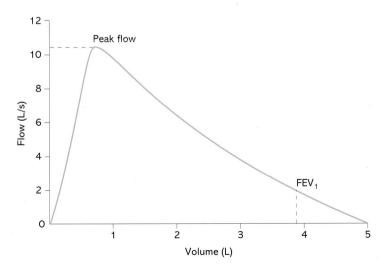

Figure 4.4 Normal flow–volume curve.

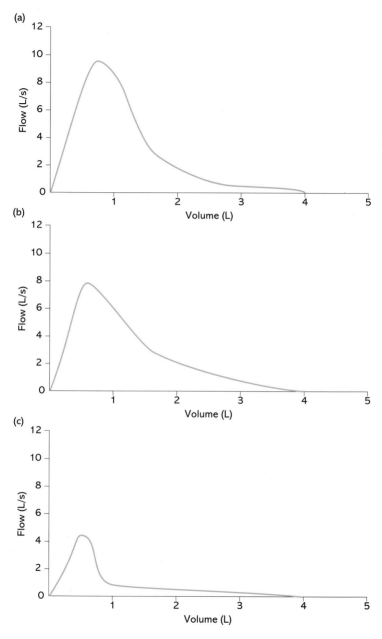

Figure 4.5 Examples of flow–volume curves. (a) Mild obstruction. (b) Moderate obstruction. (c) Severe obstruction.

The flow–volume loop can also help to identify the presence of obstruction of the large airways. The patterns of obstruction can vary with inspiration and expiration.

Lung volumes. Measurements of static lung volumes such as total lung capacity, residual volume and functional residual capacity (Figure 4.6) can be made with a body plethysmograph or by the helium dilution technique. They are used to assess the degree of overinflation and gas trapping resulting from loss of elastic recoil and collapse of the airways. It is known that dynamic overinflation occurs in COPD, particularly during exercise, and it may be an important determinant of symptoms such as breathlessness. Inspiratory capacity may be a useful surrogate for more precise measures of dynamic hyperinflation (see Figure 3.1).

The standard method for measuring static lung volumes using the helium dilution technique during rebreathing may underestimate lung volumes, particularly in patients with bullous disease, where the inspired helium does not have time to equilibrate properly in the airspaces and therefore lung volumes are underestimated. The body plethysmograph uses Boyle's law to calculate lung volumes from measurements of changes in mouth and body plethysmograph pressures

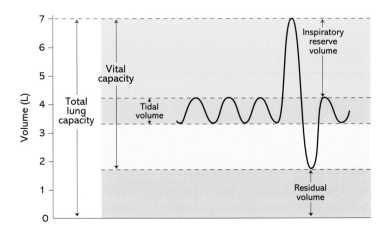

Figure 4.6 Lung volume measurements.

during gentle panting against a closed shutter. This technique measures trapped air within the thorax, thus including poorly ventilated areas, and therefore gives higher readings than the helium dilution technique in COPD. Computed tomography (CT) scans on inhalation/exhalation can also be used to measure lung volumes.

Gas transfer by the lungs can be measured using carbon monoxide as a tracer gas. Following inhalation of a small amount of carbon monoxide, some of the inhaled marker is transferred from the lungs into the pulmonary capillary blood where it binds to hemoglobin. Reductions in the concentration of carbon monoxide in the exhaled gas can therefore be used to gauge the efficiency of gas transfer within the lung. Some of the reduction in carbon monoxide level is also due to diffusion into the residual volume of the lung. Hence, values for the diffusing capacity of carbon monoxide (DLCO; TLCO in the UK) are generally corrected using helium, which diffuses into the residual volume, but is not absorbed into the pulmonary capillary blood. This technique yields the ventilated alveolar volume (V_A), which provides the carbon monoxide transfer coefficient K_{CO} (DLCO/V_A).

DLCO values are normal in asthma but below normal in many patients with COPD. Although there is a relationship between the DLCO and the extent of emphysema, the severity of the emphysema in individual patients cannot be predicted from the DLCO. Neither is a low DLCO specific for emphysema, as it can be affected by cigarette smoking, anemia and lung diseases such as pulmonary fibrosis and pulmonary thromboembolic disease. Thus a low DLCO in a patient with COPD suggests a significant degree of alveolar destruction, probably as a result of emphysema, but a normal DLCO does not exclude a diagnosis of COPD. The principal factors affecting DLCO are:

- thickness of the alveolar membrane
- capillary blood volume
- hemoglobin concentration (the test needs to be corrected for hemoglobin concentration).

The most widely used method for measuring DLCO is the single-breath technique, which measures the rate of carbon monoxide uptake during a 10-second breath hold and uses alveolar volume calculated from helium dilution during the single-breath test. This will underestimate alveolar volume in patients with severe COPD.

Arterial blood gases are important in advanced COPD to measure the degree of hypoxemia and hypercapnia and, particularly in exacerbations, to define the partial pressure of carbon dioxide in arterial blood ($PaCO_2$) and the hydrogen ion concentration or pH. The test should be performed in patients with FEV_1 less than 40% of predicted value, or when clinical signs suggest respiratory failure, right heart failure or cor pulmonale. It is essential to record the inspired oxygen concentration when reporting blood gases, and it is also important to note that it may take at least 30 minutes for a change in inspired oxygen concentration to have a full effect on the PaO_2, because alveolar gas equilibration takes a long time in COPD.

Respiratory failure is indicated by PaO_2 < 8 kPa (60 mmHg) with or without a $PaCO_2$ > 6.7 kPa (50 mmHg) while breathing air. Measurement of blood gases should be obtained by arterial puncture. Finger or ear oximeters for assessing oxygenation (percentage oxygen saturation of arterial blood, SaO_2) are less reliable but, because of their ease of use, are commonly used in clinical practice. Values of saturation ≤ 88% are indicative of the need for supplemental oxygen. Oximeters can also be used for measuring changes in oxygenation during acute exacerbations. They cannot completely replace assessment of blood gas values, however, since measurements of $PaCO_2$ are often required.

Increases in $PaCO_2$ can be compensated for by renal conservation of bicarbonate, which is a relatively slow process. Acid–base status, particularly mixed respiratory and metabolic disturbances, can be characterized by plotting values on an acid–base diagram (Figure 4.7). It can also be assessed from the arterial pH and bicarbonate.

Exercise tests. Exercise induces an increase in oxygen consumption and carbon dioxide production in skeletal muscle. Patients with COPD have the same oxygen consumption for a given workload as normal subjects. However, their dead-space ventilation is higher and so a larger minute ventilation is needed to maintain carbon dioxide at a constant level. In

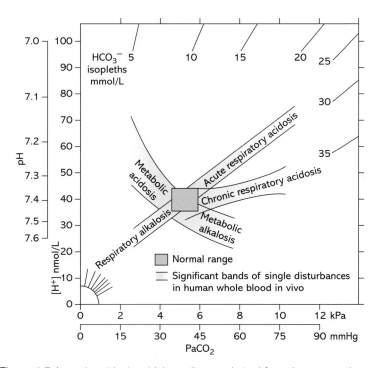

Figure 4.7 A non-logarithmic acid–base diagram derived from the measured acid–base status of patients within the five abnormal bands illustrated and of normal subjects (blue box). This plot of $PaCO_2$ against pH allows the likely acid–base disturbance and calculated bicarbonate value (obtained from the relevant isopleth) to be rapidly determined. Changes during treatment can be plotted serially for each patient. Reproduced with permission from Flenley DC. Another non-logarithmic acid–base diagram? *Lancet* 1971;1:961–5.

many patients with COPD, expiratory airflow is limited within the tidal volume range. The only way to increase minute ventilation is to increase inspiratory flow or shift the end expiratory position. Both of these maneuvers are problematic in patients with COPD and require more work from already compromised inspiratory muscles, or result in progressive overinflation, which increases both the work of breathing and symptoms.

In addition, the increased cardiac output that occurs with exercise can lead to increased perfusion of poorly ventilated areas. As a result of this ventilation–perfusion mismatch, arterial oxygenation can decline with exercise in contrast to the improvement in oxygenation that is noted in normal individuals. Decline in oxygenation with exercise is generally monitored by percutaneous oxygen saturation measurement. Exercise-induced desaturation can be an indication for supplemental oxygen therapy.

Three principal forms of exercise test are performed in COPD: progressive symptom-limited exercise, self-paced exercise and steady-state exercise. Other tests may be used in special circumstances.

Progressive symptom-limited exercise tests require patients to maintain exercise on a treadmill or a cycle until symptoms prevent them from continuing. The usual criteria for defining a maximum test are a heart rate greater than 85% of predicted or a ventilation greater than 90% predicted. The results of the test are useful, particularly when simultaneous electrocardiography (ECG) and blood pressure monitoring are performed to assess whether coexisting cardiac or psychological factors contribute to exercise limitation.

Self-paced exercise tests are easy to perform and give information on more sustained exercise, which may be more relevant to performance in daily life. The 6-minute walk is the most commonly used test, with a coefficient of variation of around 8%. There may, however, be a learning effect that influences the result of repeated tests. This test is only useful in patients with moderately severe COPD (FEV_1 < 1.5 liters) who would be expected to have an exercise tolerance of less than 600 meters in 6 minutes. There is only a weak relationship between walking distance and FEV_1. The shuttle walking test is an alternative in which the patient performs a paced walk between two points 10 meters apart (a shuttle). The pace of the walk is increased at regular intervals, dictated by bleeps on a tape recording, until the patient is forced to stop because of breathlessness. The number of completed shuttles is recorded.

Steady-state exercise tests require exercise at a sustainable percentage of maximum capacity for 3–6 minutes while blood gases are measured, enabling calculation of the dead space:tidal volume ratio (V_D:V_T) and the passage through the lungs without oxygenation (shunt). This assessment is seldom required in patients with COPD.

Other more complex tests, such as assessing the lung pressure–volume curve, are difficult to undertake, requiring measurement of esophageal pressure with an esophageal balloon, and are not part of the routine assessment, but may be necessary in special circumstances. Measurements of small airways function, such as the nitrogen washout test, helium and air flow–volume loops and frequency dependency of compliance (the dependence of lung compliance on respiratory frequency), have poor reproducibility in patients with COPD. Although they can differentiate smokers from non-smokers, they are not useful in predicting which smokers will develop COPD and thus are not used in routine practice.

Assessment of breathlessness

Improvement in symptoms, particularly breathlessness, is one of the important goals of treatment in COPD. Although breathlessness is a subjective feature, it should be quantified. There are several scales for assessing breathlessness objectively (see Chapter 3).

The MRC Dyspnea Scale (see Table 3.2) allows patients to rate their breathlessness according to the activity that induces it. It is graded from 0 to 5 and is easy to use, but it is insensitive to change and may be more valuable as a baseline assessment than as a means of measuring the effect of treatment.

The oxygen-cost diagram is more sensitive to change than the MRC scale. It allows the patient to place a mark on a 10-cm line to represent the point beyond which they become breathless (Figure 4.8), and the distance in centimeters from the zero point can be used to obtain a score. Other scales allow quantification of the breathlessness according to the intensity of the sensation. The Borg Scale (Table 3.1) is useful for measuring short-term changes in intensity of breathlessness during a particular task. It is sensitive and reproducible. A simple analog scale is another method of allowing patients to rate the intensity of their breathlessness. As with the oxygen-cost diagram, a 10-cm line is drawn on a page and the patient then marks on the line how intense their breathlessness is, from 0 centimeters, not at all, to 10 cm, intensely breathless. The score is the distance along the line that the patient has marked.

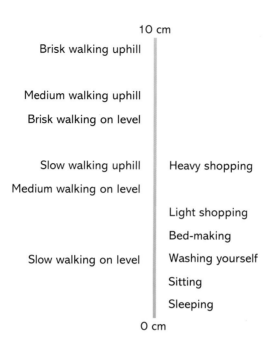

Figure 4.8 Oxygen-cost diagram.

Health status

Health status, or quality of life, is a measure of the impact of disease on daily life and well-being. COPD has a marked effect on health status, particularly owing to breathlessness limiting exercise, reducing expectation, limiting daily activity, restricting social activities, disturbing mood and impairing well-being. There are several questionnaires available for the measurement of health status, which are mainly used in hospital rehabilitation programs and in research. The Chronic Respiratory Disease Index Questionnaire is sensitive to change but is very time-consuming and requires training to administer properly. The St George's Respiratory Questionnaire is a self-completed questionnaire with three components that give a total score of overall health status: symptoms, measuring distress due to respiratory symptoms; activity, measuring disturbance of daily activities; and impact, which measures psychosocial function. The Breathing Problems Questionnaire is a similar self-completed questionnaire, which is easy to complete but relatively insensitive to change. The St George's Respiratory Questionnaire has been most validated in COPD. Although there is a relationship between the St George's questionnaire and FEV_1 value as a percentage of predicted, the relationship is rather poor. From various studies it is clear that there can be treatment-related improvement in the St George's health status without any improvement in FEV_1. The threshold of clinical improvement is a change of four units in the St George's questionnaire. Exacerbations of COPD have a clear detrimental effect on health status. These questionnaires are not as yet used in clinical practice.

Sleep studies

Patients with COPD become increasingly hypoxemic during sleep, particularly during rapid eye movement (REM) sleep. There is no evidence that measurement of nocturnal hypoxemia provides any further prognostic or clinically useful information in the assessment of patients with COPD unless coexisting sleep apnea syndrome is suspected. Individuals who desaturate during the night may, however, be candidates for oxygen therapy.

Other assessments

Polycythemia. In patients with severe COPD, identifying polycythemia is important since it predisposes to vascular events. Polycythemia should be suspected when the hematocrit is more than 47% in women and more than 52% in men, and/or the hemoglobin is greater than 16 g/dL in women and greater than 18 g/dL in men, provided other causes of spurious polycythemia due to decreased plasma volume, such as occurs with dehydration, can be excluded.

α_1-antitrypsin deficiency screening. In patients younger than 45 years who develop COPD and/or have a strong family history of the disease, levels of α_1-antitrypsin should be measured.

Electrocardiography. Routine ECG is not required in the assessment of patients with COPD, and is an insensitive technique in the diagnosis of cor pulmonale.

Key points – lung function tests

- Spirometry is the most important measurement in COPD and is essential for diagnosis. Forced expiratory volume in 1 second (FEV_1) and forced vital capacity (FVC) are recorded in absolute values (liters) and also as a percentage of the predicted values for the individual depending on age, height, gender and ethnic origin.
- An FEV_1 over 80% of the predicted value is considered to be normal.
- Airflow obstruction is defined as an FEV_1 below 80% of the predicted value and an FEV_1:FVC ratio < 70%.
- A standardized technique must be employed in assessing spirometry. It is critical that the expiratory flow trace reaches a plateau, proving that the patient has blown to FVC.
- Reversibility testing to bronchodilators is useful in differential diagnosis to distinguish those with marked reversibility, indictative of asthma.
- There is no standard assessment of reversibility; generally, however, an improvement in FEV_1 by both 200 mL and 15% over the baseline is interpreted as a positive result.
- Peak expiratory flow rate is not the best assessment of airway obstruction in COPD and may underestimate the degree of airway obstruction.
- Further tests of lung volumes and DLCO may be helpful in some cases.

Key references

Borg G. Psychophysical basis of perceived exertion. *Med Sci Sports Exerc* 1982;84:377–81.

British Thoracic Society Guidelines for the management of chronic obstructive pulmonary disease. *Thorax* 1997;52(suppl 5):S1–S28.

Gibson GJ, MacNee W. Chronic obstructive pulmonary disease: investigations and assessment of severity. *Eur Respir Monogr* 1998;7:25–40.

Global Initiative for Chronic Obstructive Lung Disease. Assessment. In: *Global Strategy for the Diagnosis, Management, and Prevention of Chronic Obstructive Pulmonary Disease. NHLBI/WHO Workshop Report.* National Heart, Lung, and Blood Institute (USA), World Health Organization: 2001, updated 2003:27–44. www.goldcopd.com

Guyatt GH, Berman LB, Townsend M et al. A measure of quality of life for clinical trials in chronic lung disease. *Thorax* 1987; 42:773–8.

Jones PW, Quirk FH, Baveystock CM, Littlejohns P. A self-complete measure for chronic airflow limitation: the St. George's questionnaire. *Am Rev Respir Dis* 1992;147:832–8.

McGavin CR, Artvinli M, Naoe H. Dyspnoea, disability and distance walked: a comparison of estimates of exercise performance in respiratory disease. *BMJ* 1978;2:241–3.

Noseda A, Carpeiaux JP, Schmerber J. Dyspnoea assessed by visual analogue scale in patients with obstructive lung disease during progressive and high intensity exercise. *Thorax* 1992;47:363–8.

Pauwels R, Buist AS, Calverley PM et al. The GOLD Scientific Committee. Global strategy for the diagnosis, management, and prevention of chronic obstructive pulmonary disease. NHLBI/WHO Global Initiative for Chronic Obstructive Lung Disease (GOLD) Workshop summary. *Am J Respir Crit Care Med* 2001;163:1256–76.

Singh SJ, Morgan MDL, Scott SC et al. The development of the shuttle walking test of disability in patients with chronic airway obstruction. *Thorax* 1992:47:1019–24.

There are no features specific for COPD on a plain posterior-anterior chest radiograph. The features usually described are those of severe emphysema. However, there may be no abnormalities, even in patients with very appreciable disability. Recent improvements in imaging techniques, particularly the advent of computed tomography (CT) and, more recently, high-resolution computed tomography (HRCT), have provided more sensitive means of diagnosing emphysema in life.

Plain chest radiography

The most reliable radiographic signs of emphysema can be classified by their causes of overinflation, vascular changes and bullae.

Overinflation of the lungs results in the following radiographic features:
- a low, flattened diaphragm (Figure 5.1); the diaphragm is abnormally low if the border of the diaphragm in the midclavicular

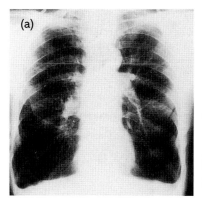 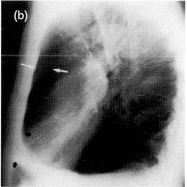

Figure 5.1 Plain chest radiographs of generalized emphysema particularly affecting the lower zones. (a) Posterior-anterior radiograph showing a low, flat diaphragm (below the anterior ends of the seventh ribs), obtuse costophrenic angles and reduced vessel markings in lower zones, which are transradiant. (b) Lateral radiograph showing a low, flat and inverted diaphragm and widened retrosternal transradiancy (white arrows) that approaches the diaphragm inferiorly (black arrows).

line is at or below the anterior end of the seventh rib, and is
flattened if the perpendicular height from a line drawn between the
costal and cardiophrenic angles to the border of the diaphragm is
less than 1.5 cm
- increased retrosternal airspace, visible on the lateral film at a point
  3 cm below the manubrium when the horizontal distance from the
  posterior surface of the aorta to the sternum exceeds 4.5 cm
- an obtuse costophrenic angle on the posterior-anterior or lateral
  chest radiograph
- an inferior margin of the retrosternal airspace 3 cm or less from the
  anterior aspect of the diaphragm.

Vascular changes associated with emphysema result from loss of
alveolar walls and are shown on the plain chest radiograph by:
- a reduction in the size and number of pulmonary vessels, particularly
  at the periphery of the lung
- vessel distortion, producing increased branching angles, excess
  straightening or bowing of vessels
- areas of transradiancy.

Assessment of the vascular loss in emphysema clearly depends on the
quality of the radiograph. A generally increased transradiancy may
simply be due to overexposure. Focal areas of transradiancy
surrounded by hairline walls represent bullae.

The development of right ventricular hypertrophy produces non-
specific cardiac enlargement on the plain chest radiograph. Pulmonary
hypertension can be assessed from the plain chest radiograph by
measuring the width of the right descending pulmonary artery,
measured just below the right hilum, where the borders of the artery
are delineated against the air in the lungs laterally and the right main
stem bronchus medially. The upper limit of the normal range of the
width of the artery in this area is 16 mm in males and 15 mm in
females. This increase in pulmonary artery size is often associated with
a rapid diminution of the size of the vessels as they branch into the
pulmonary periphery. Although these measurements can be used to
detect the presence or absence of pulmonary hypertension, they cannot
accurately predict the level of the pulmonary artery pressure.

Computed tomography

CT scanning has been used to detect and quantify emphysema. Techniques can be divided into those that use visual assessment of low-density areas on the CT scan, which can be either semiquantitative or quantitative, or those which use CT lung density to quantify areas of low X-ray attenuation. These two techniques are usually employed to measure macroscopic or microscopic emphysema, respectively.

A visual assessment of emphysema on CT scanning (Figure 5.2) reveals:

- areas of low attenuation without obvious margins or walls
- attenuation and pruning of the vascular tree
- abnormal vascular configurations.

The sign that correlates best with areas of macroscopic emphysema is an area of low attenuation. Visual inspection of the CT scan can locate areas of macroscopic emphysema, although a visual assessment of the extent of macroscopic emphysema is insensitive and subjective, with a high intra- and inter-observer variability.

It is possible to distinguish the various types of emphysema by means of HRCT, particularly when the changes are not severe. The distinction depends on the distribution of the lesions: those of centrilobular emphysema are patchy and prominent in the upper zones, whereas those of panlobular emphysema are diffuse throughout the lung zones.

CT measurement of lung density in terms of Hounsfield units (a scale of X-ray attenuation where bone = +1000 HU, water is zero and air is –1000 HU) provides a more quantitative way of measuring emphysema, particularly at the microscopic level (Figure 5.3).

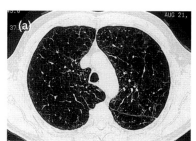
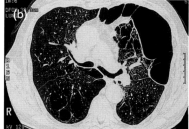

Figure 5.2 High-resolution CT scans of the lungs. (a) Diffuse panlobular emphysema. (b) More patchy centrilobular emphysema with bullae.

A quantitative approach to assessing macroscopic emphysema has been taken by highlighting picture elements, or pixels, within the lung fields in a predetermined low density range, between –910 and –1000 Hounsfield units, the 'density mask' technique.

If CT scanning is to be used to measure microscopic emphysema, care should be taken to standardize the scanning conditions, particularly the lung volume, and to calibrate the CT scanner, since these factors affect CT lung density. These techniques have not, as yet, been sufficiently standardized for use in clinical practice, but density measurements have been shown to correlate with morphometric measurements of distal airspace size in resected lungs.

Whether a bulla is detected on a chest X-ray depends on its size and the degree to which it is obscured by overlying lung. CT scanning is much more sensitive than plain chest radiography in detecting bullae and can be used to determine their number, size and position.

Echocardiography

Echocardiography has been used to assess the right ventricle and for detection of pulmonary hypertension in COPD. However, overinflation of the chest increases the retrosternal airspace, which therefore transmits sound waves poorly, making echocardiography difficult in patients with COPD. Nevertheless, an adequate examination can be achieved in 65–85% of patients with COPD.

Two-dimensional echocardiography has been used in the investigation of right ventricular dimensions and is superior to clinical methods since it shows reasonable correlations between pulmonary artery pressure and various right ventricular dimensions.

Pulsed-wave Doppler echocardiography has been used to assess the ejection flow dynamics of the right ventricle in patients with pulmonary hypertension. The parameters measured include acceleration time (in milliseconds), defined as the time between the onset of ejection to peak velocity; right ventricular pre-ejection time (in milliseconds), the interval from the Q wave of the ECG to the beginning of the forward flow; and right ventricular ejection time (in milliseconds), the interval between the onset and termination of flow in the right ventricular outflow tract. Although the pulsed-wave Doppler technique is useful in differentiating

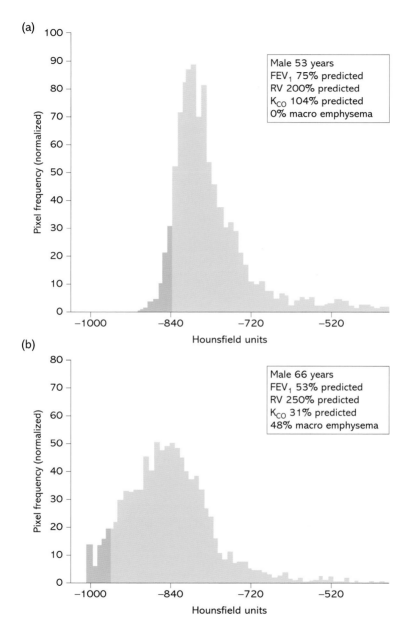

Figure 5.3 (a) Density histogram for a subject with no emphysema. (b) Density histogram for a patient with severe emphysema. The darker area represents the lowest 5% of the distribution.

patients with an elevated pulmonary arterial pressure from those with normal pulmonary arterial pressure, it is not as accurate as the continuous-wave Doppler technique in assessing pulmonary arterial pressure.

The best technique for non-invasive evaluation of pulmonary arterial pressure is continuous-wave Doppler echocardiography; the tricuspid gradient thus assessed can be used to calculate the right ventricular systolic pressure. The technique estimates the pressure gradient across the regurgitant jet recorded by Doppler ultrasound. The maximum velocity of the regurgitant jet is measured from the continuous-wave Doppler recordings, and the simplified Bernoulli equation is used to calculate the maximum pressure gradient between the right ventricle and the right atrium as:

$$P_{RV} - P_{RA} = 4v^2$$

where P_{RV} and P_{RA} are the right ventricular and right atrial pressures and v is the maximum velocity. The right atrial pressure is estimated from clinical examination of the jugular venous pressure. There is still debate as to whether this technique is sensitive and reproducible enough to monitor longitudinal changes in pulmonary arterial pressure and the effects of therapeutic interventions, particularly in patients with COPD.

Key points – imaging

- No features on a plain chest radiograph are specific for COPD; the features usually described are those of severe emphysema. However, there may be no abnormality even in patients with marked disability.
- Computerized tomography (CT) can be used to quantify emphysema, either by visual assessment of high-resolution scanning or by CT lung density measurements.
- CT scanning is the best way to detect and assess bullous disease.
- Echocardiography, particularly continuous-wave Doppler echocardiography, can be used to assess pulmonary arterial pressure in patients with COPD.

Key references

Gould GA, MacNee W, McLean A et al. CT measurements of lung density in life can quantitate distal airspace enlargement – an essential defining feature of human emphysema. *Am Rev Respir Dis* 1988;137:380–92.

Gould GA, Redpath AT, Ryan M et al. Parenchymal emphysema measured by CT lung density correlates with lung function in patients with bullous disease. *Eur Respir J* 1993;6:698–704.

MacNee W. Chronic bronchitis and emphysema. In: Seaton A, Seaton D, Leitch AG, eds. *Crofton and Douglas's Respiratory Diseases 1*. Oxford: Blackwell Science, 2000:616–95.

O'Brien C, Guest PJ, Hill SL, Stockley RA. Physiological and radiological characterization of patients diagnosed with chronic obstructive pulmonary disease in primary care. *Thorax* 2000;55: 635–42.

6 Smoking cessation

Cigarette smoking is the single most important factor in the development of COPD. Smoking cessation is therefore the single most important therapeutic intervention. The earlier a smoker quits, the more advantages accrue.

The majority (over 85%) of cigarette smokers are addicted to nicotine and experience a well-defined withdrawal syndrome following cessation (Table 6.1). These symptoms peak in the first few days following cessation and gradually decrease after 2–3 weeks. Episodes of craving, which may be intense, may recur for many years; they are often initiated by environmental or behavioral cues associated with smoking. It is important that smokers be informed that these cravings will subside with or without relapse to smoking.

Smoking should not be regarded as a lifestyle choice, but, owing to the addiction, as a primary disease entity in itself. Smoking cessation is

TABLE 6.1

Withdrawal syndrome following smoking cessation, defined in the _DSM-IV_

- Dysphoric or depressed mood
- Insomnia
- Irritability, frustration or anger
- Anxiety
- Difficulty concentrating
- Restlessness
- Decreased heart rate
- Increased appetite or weight gain
- Craving to smoke*

*Not included in _DSM-IV_ for 'logical reasons' but a characteristic of the syndrome
DSM-IV, Diagnostic and Statistical Manual of Mental Disorders of the American Psychiatric Association, 4th edn

thus not simply a matter of personal choice, but is a legitimate therapeutic intervention.

Recent data indicate that smokers differ in their biological propensity to become smokers and that genetic factors may affect their ability to quit. Therapeutic interventions targeted at individual smokers' susceptibilities are currently under intensive investigation. Available therapies can nevertheless help a substantial minority of smokers to quit.

Among adult smokers, approximately 70% wish to stop smoking, and as many as 45% make a serious attempt in each year. Despite this, only 2% of smokers successfully quit spontaneously in a year. Simple physician advice to quit can increase these rates to 5–6%. Additional behavioral support as well as pharmacological therapy can further increase quit rates. Current recommendations, therefore, are that all physicians establish smoking status as a 'vital sign' at every visit and that appropriate smoking intervention be undertaken (Figure 6.1). These steps ensure that smokers receive maximum encouragement to quit.

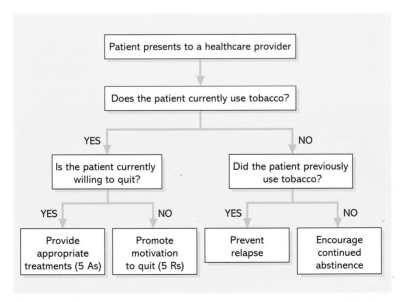

Figure 6.1 Brief antismoking intervention to be undertaken at every visit to the healthcare provider.

- Brief interventions should be implemented in all practices.
- Intensive interventions are appropriate for many COPD patients. Each practitioner caring for COPD patients should have the option of referring patients for intensive intervention.
- Systems approaches to ensure smoking cessation intervention is integrated into each practice and fully supported by the healthcare system.

Brief interventions

Brief interventions can be highly effective for many smokers. The five As (Table 6.2) provide key steps for a brief intervention that can be accomplished within a few minutes and can be tailored to the needs of each smoker.

Smokers not yet ready to quit should be provided with a brief intervention to increase motivation. This should be sympathetic and non-confrontational and should provide patient-specific information. The five Rs can provide guidance in this respect (Table 6.3). The patient should also understand that the physician is working in their best interest and will be prepared to offer appropriate smoking cessation counseling when the patient is ready.

TABLE 6.2

The five As for physician intervention

- **Ask:** Implement a system that ensures that tobacco use is queried and documented for *every* patient at *every* clinic visit

- **Advise:** In a clear, strong and personalized manner, urge all tobacco users to quit

- **Assess:** Ask every tobacco user if he or she is willing to attempt to quit at this time (e.g., within the next 30 days)

- **Assist:** Help the patient make a quit plan, provide practical counseling and intra-treatment social support, help the patient obtain extra-treatment social support, recommend use of approved pharmacotherapy (except in special circumstances) and provide supplementary materials

- **Arrange:** Schedule follow-up contact, either in person or by telephone

TABLE 6.3

The five Rs for smoker motivation

- **Relevance**: Personalize the reasons to quit. This may include issues in addition to COPD

- **Risks**: – *Acute*: dyspnea, cough, exacerbations, increased carbon monoxide levels

  – *Chronic*: COPD progression, cancer, cardiovascular disease, osteoporosis, peptic ulcer

  – *Environmental*: disease risk to spouse, household members, increased risk of smoking and of disease in children

- **Rewards**: – Improved health

  – Improved self-image, sense of taste and smell

  – Saves money

  – Example for children

- **Roadblocks**: – Withdrawal symptoms

  – Fear of failure

  – Weight gain

  – Lack of support

  – Depression

  – Enjoyment of tobacco

- **Repetition**: Most smokers make several quit attempts before achieving long-term abstinence; smoking can be regarded as a chronic relapsing condition, but prolonged remissions are possible

Every smoker ready to attempt to quit should be offered the highest probability of success. Behavioral support, pharmacological treatment and follow-up all contribute to success.

Behavioral support. Data show clearly that the more behavioral support offered, the more likely a smoker is to quit. Many smokers, however, will not attend intensive behavioral programs. Brief behavioral help is therefore appropriate for most individuals. There are a number of approaches, shown in Table 6.4.

Pharmacological treatment. All smokers making a serious attempt to quit should be offered pharmacological treatment (in the absence of contraindications). Treatment with first-line medicines for smoking cessation approximately doubles quit rates. Second-line treatments should be considered for smokers who have failed first-line treatment.

First-line treatments for smoking cessation include nicotine replacement therapy and bupropion (recommended international non-

TABLE 6.4

Behavioral support for smokers trying to quit

Help establish a quit plan

- Set a quit date (ideally within 2 weeks)
- Tell family and friends
- Anticipate challenges
- Remove tobacco products

Counseling

- Be aware that abstinence is essential (most smokers who smoke at all after the quit date will relapse to the previous habit)
- Utilize experience from previous quit attempts
- Anticipate challenges
- Avoid alcohol (the most frequent relapses occur with concurrent alcohol)
- Consider the effect of other smokers in the household (supportive, obstructive, prepared to quit too?)

Encourage other support

- Enlist family, friends and co-workers to assist
- Find support groups

Provide educational materials

- Should be available in every clinician's office. Many are available through a variety of agencies

proprietary name amfebutamone; bupropion is the US generic and former British approved name).

Nicotine replacement is available in several formulations: nicotine polacrilex gum, transdermal nicotine systems, nicotine inhaler, nicotine nasal spray and nicotine lozenges. Several other formulations are currently under investigation. All are similar in efficacy but differ in clinical use (Table 6.5).

The use of nicotine replacement therapy for smoking cessation is based on the pharmacokinetics of nicotine as a psychoactive drug. The 'hit' associated with nicotine depends on both the amount of nicotine that reaches the brain and the rate of rise in the concentration. The peaks not only provide the psychoactive effect of nicotine but contribute to both the psychological and the biological reinforcing mechanisms leading to addiction. Withdrawal symptoms are believed to develop when nicotine levels fall below a certain threshold (Figure 6.2). This generally occurs several hours after the last cigarette, as nicotine has a half-life on the order of hours in most individuals. The concept behind nicotine replacement therapy, therefore, is to provide a steady-state level that can protect against the symptoms of withdrawal without providing the reinforcement that contributes to addiction.

Currently available nicotine formulations provide only partial nicotine replacement for most smokers, and none completely prevents withdrawal symptoms, but they do reduce them. More importantly, nicotine replacement therapies increase quit rates. The general strategy for their use is to establish a quit day and to start nicotine replacement on that day. Therapy is then continued for 10 weeks to 6 months. There are individual differences in preference for the various formulations, allowing the physician some choice in individualizing therapy. The various formulations also have different pharmacokinetics. This is likely to affect their potential to sustain addiction; many individuals have substituted nicotine gum for cigarettes, but remained addicted. It is generally considered, however, that the health hazards associated with the gum are dramatically less than those associated with smoking.

Because the available formulations generally provide incomplete nicotine replacement, there is some possibility for combination therapy.

TABLE 6.5

Nicotine delivery systems

Formulation, time to onset, blood level*	Administration
Cigarette, 10 min, 40 ng/mL	
–	–
Patch, 500 min, 20 ng/mL**	
A reservoir containing nicotine is applied directly to the skin. Because of its volatility and lipid solubility, nicotine penetrates the skin and is absorbed into capillary blood	Apply to a normal, non-hairy area of skin. Rotate applications
Gum, 30 min, 20 ng/mL	
Nicotine is bound to a polacrilex resin and is released by chewing. It must be absorbed into capillary blood through the buccal mucosa. Swallowed nicotine can irritate the stomach, but is largely metabolized by the liver	Gum must be chewed to release nicotine; release rate parallels chewing rate. Swallowing prevents effective absorption. Acid in the mouth (e.g. from coffee or orange juice) interferes with absorption. Number of pieces of gum can be altered to suit the individual – general range is 5–30 pieces/day
Inhaler, 30 min, 7 ng/mL	
A mouthpiece is connected to a cartridge containing 10 mg nicotine adsorbed onto a porous support. Approximately 4 mg nicotine can be released and 2 mg absorbed (through the oral mucosa or lower respiratory tract) by inhalation through the device	6–8 cartridges/day recommended as initial therapy
Nasal spray, 10 min, 20 ng/mL	
Nicotine solution (10 mg/mL) is atomized in a spray	One spray into each nostril for each dose. Dosing can be adjusted to suit the individual; generally at least 8 doses/day and up to 2 doses/hour are recommended

* Blood levels for repeated dosing formulations vary with dosing
** The pharmacokinetics of the various transdermal patches differ

Dose[†]	Advantages	Disadvantages
–	–	Health hazard
7, 14, 21 mg/day (Nicoderm, Habitrol, Niquitin, Nicotinell) 11, 22 mg/day (Prostep) 5, 10, 15 mg/16 h (Nicotrol, Nicorette)	Constant and simple administration. Overnight administration can reduce intensity of craving and withdrawal symptoms on waking	Local skin irritation. Overnight administration sometimes associated with sleep disturbance and intense dreaming
2 and 4 mg/piece	Dose and regimen can be changed to suit the individual	Local problems may result from chewing (e.g. jaw pain, denture problems etc.) or from nicotine (e.g. hiccoughs, gastrointestinal distress)
4 mg/cartridge	Dose and regimen can be individualized	Locally irritating
Each actuation delivers 0.5 mg nicotine to one nostril (2 sprays deliver total dose of 1 mg nicotine)	Dose and regimen can be timed to suit the individual	Locally irritating. Nasal symptoms very common but seldom preclude administration. Nasal congestion can disrupt absorption.

[†] Dose refers to the amount of nicotine nominally absorbed over the duration of administration; the various systems contain different amounts of residual nicotine after use

Several reports suggest that this can offer benefits, although it is an off-label use.

Bupropion is the only non-nicotine agent approved for smoking cessation. It acts directly on the central nervous system, and is in use as an antidepressant. It approximately doubles quit rates, and may be particularly effective in individuals with a prior history of depression. Bupropion and nicotine replacement therapy can be used in combination. Bupropion is generally started one week before the quit day so that adequate blood levels can be achieved. The usual initial dose is 150 mg once a day, increased to twice a day after three days if tolerated. Bupropion should not be used in individuals at risk of seizures or with a history of bulimia or anorexia, and should not be additionally prescribed for those who are currently receiving bupropion for the treatment of depression.

Second-line therapies. Two second-line treatments are available, clonidine and nortriptyline. Clonidine has been evaluated in several

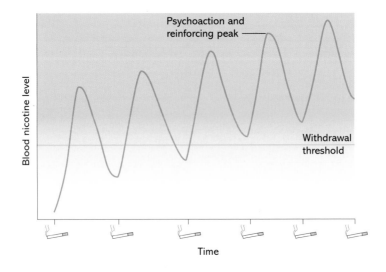

Figure 6.2 Peaks in nicotine blood level provide the psychoactive effect and contribute to the psychological and biological reinforcing mechanisms leading to addiction. Withdrawal symptoms are believed to develop when nicotine levels fall below a certain threshold.

clinical trials, and, although it is not approved and the individual trials did not consistently show statistically significant benefits, a meta-analysis supports its use. The physician comfortable with this medication can consider it an aid to smoking cessation.

The antidepressant nortriptyline has also been evaluated in three clinical trials, which showed clinical efficacy. This agent is available as an antidepressant and can therefore be used off-label for smoking cessation by physicians comfortable with its use.

Follow-up evaluations. Success in smoking cessation is closely linked to follow-up. All smokers making a serious quit attempt should therefore be offered follow-up assessment. Such assessments can deal with specific problems related to cessation and medication use, and can provide behavioral support. Follow-up 1–2 weeks after the quit day is generally recommended. Additional follow-ups can also be beneficial.

Intensive interventions

Intensive interventions are more elaborate than the brief interventions described above. Generally speaking, they require trained counselors and can be conducted either as individual or group sessions. Most often multiple sessions are conducted. Only a minority of smokers referred for intensive programs will attend. Such programs can, however, offer

Key points – smoking cessation

- Smoking should be regarded as a primary chronic relapsing disease.
- All serious attempts to quit should be maximally supported with behavioral and pharmacologic interventions.
- Repeated efforts by the physician are required to provide sufficient motivation for a quit attempt.
- Relapses are common, and should engender repeated attempts.
- Smoking cessation activities should be an integrated part of every medical practice.

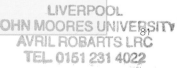

an important support for many smokers, and every practitioner should be able to refer patients for intensive intervention.

Systems approaches

Cigarette smoking should be regarded as a primary disease, and its treatment should be integrated into each healthcare system. This includes adequate training of personnel to interview patients for smoking status as a 'vital sign'. The healthcare system should provide adequate support for smoking cessation efforts. Personnel at all levels should be active participants in smoking cessation interventions.

Key references

Daughton D, Susman J, Sitorius M et al. Transdermal nicotine therapy and primary care: Importance of counseling, demographic and patient selection factors on one-year quit rates. The Nebraska Primary Practice Smoking Cessation Trial Group. *Arch Fam Med* 1998;7:425–30.

Fiore MC. US public health service clinical practice guideline: treating tobacco use and dependence. *Respir Care* 2000;45:1200–62.

Fiore MC, Bailey WC, Cohen SJ. *Smoking cessation. Guideline technical report no. 18.* Rockville, MD: US Dept of Health and Human Services, Public Health Service, Agency for Health Care Policy and Research. Publication No. AHCPR 97-No4, October 1997.

Jorenby DE, Leischow SJ, Nides MA et al. A controlled trial of sustained-release bupropion, a nicotine patch, or both for smoking cessation. *New Engl J Med* 1999;340:685–91.

Rennard SI, Daughton DM. Cigarette smoking and disease. In: Fishman A, Elias J, Fishman J et al., eds. *Pulmonary Diseases and Disorders*. New York: McGraw–Hill, 1998:697–708.

Schwartz JL. *Review and evaluation of smoking cessation methods: the United States and Canada, 1978–1985.* NIH Publication No. 87-2940, 1987:1125–56.

Transdermal Nicotine Study Group. Transdermal nicotine for smoking cessation. Six-month results from two multicenter controlled clinical trials. *JAMA* 1991;266:3133–8.

West R, Shiffman S. *Fast Facts – Smoking Cessation*. Oxford: Health Press, 2004.

7 Therapy in stable disease

Pharmacological treatment: bronchodilators

Rationale and physiology of benefit. Bronchodilators are the first-line treatment for patients with COPD. It may seem paradoxical that COPD, a disease which, by definition, has at best limited reversibility, is treated with bronchodilators as first-line therapy. However, even small improvements in airflow can mean a significant improvement for COPD patients. Most people have some degree of airway smooth muscle tone, including patients with COPD. Thus, normal individuals will often experience a very modest improvement in airflow when given a bronchodilator. Sedentary normal individuals seldom notice any ease in breathing as a result. Patients with COPD, however, for whom the cost of breathing is substantially greater, especially on exercising, often notice significant improvements in the ease with which they breathe with even modest improvements in airflow.

Even in the absence of measurable improvements in airflow, moreover, patients with COPD may still derive benefit from bronchodilators. The likely explanation is that airflow in COPD patients is not only compromised, but is irregularly compromised. As a result, the rate at which different portions of the lung empty during exhalation is variable. With increasing respiratory rate, the areas most severely affected become hyperinflated (see Chapter 2). Subtle improvements in airflow, which result in better matching of the rates with which various portions of the lung empty, probably have an important effect on lung volumes, particularly with increasing respiratory rates, even if total airflow is relatively unaffected. This can lead to a gratifying apparent paradox in which a patient has significant clinical improvement in dyspnea on exertion in the absence of any measurable improvement in FEV_1 at rest.

Clinical monitoring. In view of the above, all patients with COPD should be treated initially and aggressively with bronchodilators to control symptoms. Their response should be monitored with objective

83

measures of airflow and on the basis of clinical outcomes such as symptoms and performance. All of these can aid the clinician in the care of the patient. Adequate assessment of clinical response may require exercise challenge. It is common for patients with COPD to restrict their level of activity progressively as the disease worsens (see page 29). This reduces dyspnea, but at the cost of an increasingly sedentary existence. Administration of bronchodilators is often insufficient by itself to treat such patients. Usually, improvements in physiological function can benefit the patient only if the bronchodilator treatment is used together with an aggressive rehabilitation program (see below). Thus, while bronchodilators form first-line therapy in COPD, their successful use requires their integration into an appropriate management plan, such as that suggested in the GOLD guidelines (Table 7.1).

In mild COPD ($FEV_1 \geq 80\%$ predicted), patients are unlikely to experience dyspnea. If dyspnea does develop, short-acting bronchodilators can be given on an as-needed basis. Since dyspnea is most likely to develop following exercise, it may be prudent to give bronchodilators prior to exertion in order to facilitate a greater level of activity rather than to administer them following exertion. Long-acting bronchodilators may be advantageous to maintain high levels of activity.

For patients with moderate COPD, regular treatment with one or more bronchodilators is recommended. Long-acting bronchodilators are appealing, as optimizing airflow for as long as possible throughout the day and night seems advantageous in maximizing performance ability. As noted above, this treatment should be integrated into an exercise and/or rehabilitation program. Inhaled glucocorticoids can be considered. They are most likely to be of benefit as the disease worsens and exacerbation frequency increases.

Bronchodilator classes. There are three main classes of bronchodilators: β-agonists, anticholinergics and theophylline (Figure 7.1). Both short-acting and long-acting agents or formulations are available (or will be available) in all three classes.

β-agonists act as bronchodilators on the β_2 subclass of β-agonist receptors in airway smooth muscle by increasing cyclic adenosine

TABLE 7.1

GOLD guidelines for treatment of stable COPD

Stage	Characteristics	Recommended treatment
0: At risk	Chronic symptoms (cough, sputum) Known exposure to risk factor(s) Normal spirometry	Avoidance of risk factor(s) Influenza vaccination Education of patients as to how and when to use their treatments Review of treatments prescribed for other conditions Avoidance of β-blocking agents (including eye-drop formulations)
I: Mild COPD	$FEV_1:FVC < 70\%$ $FEV_1 \geq 80\%$ predicted With or without symptoms	As above, *plus* Short-acting bronchodilator when needed
II: Moderate	$FEV_1:FVC < 70\%$ $50\% \leq FEV_1 < 80\%$ predicted With or without symptoms	As above, *plus* Regular treatment with one or more long-acting bronchodilators Rehabilitation
III: Severe	$FEV_1:FVC < 70\%$ $30\% \leq FEV_1 < 50\%$ predicted With or without symptoms	As above, *plus* Inhaled glucocorticoids if repeated exacerbations
IV: Very severe	$FEV_1:FVC < 70\%$ $FEV_1 < 30\%$ predicted or presence of respiratory failure or right heart failure	As above, *plus* Long-term oxygen therapy if chronic respiratory failure present Consider surgical treatments

Adapted from GOLD Workshop Report Executive Summary, April 2003 (www.goldcopd.com)

monophosphate (cAMP) levels and thus decreasing airway smooth muscle tone. β-agonists can act on β-receptors on other cell types as well. By relaxing vascular smooth muscle, they can increase blood flow

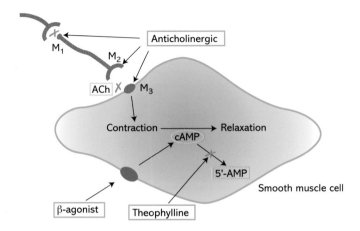

Figure 7.1 Mechanisms of action of bronchodilators. Anticholinergics block muscarinic receptors so that acetylcholine is unable to act upon them; β-agonists increase levels of cAMP; theophylline blocks conversion of cAMP to 5'-AMP. M_1, M_2 and M_3 are three distinct types of muscarinic cholinergic receptors. ACh, acetylcholine; AMP, adenosine monophosphate; cAMP, cyclic AMP.

to relatively poorly ventilated areas and may thus cause a reduction in oxygenation in some settings. Effects on airway epithelial cells and inflammatory cells may be beneficial (see below), but the clinical importance of all these non-bronchodilator effects remains uncertain.

A variety of β-agonists are available in a number of formulations (Table 7.2). They fall roughly into two classes, short-acting and long-acting. Most of the β-agonists commonly in use are relatively selective for the $β_2$-receptor subtype. As a result, they have relatively fewer cardiac side effects than do older, non-selective β-agonists such as isoproterenol, as these act on the heart primarily through $β_1$-receptors. However, because the heart has some $β_2$-receptors, no selective agent will be entirely free of cardiac effects.

Short-acting β-agonists. Most short-acting β-agonists have a relatively rapid onset of action, achieving measurable bronchodilation within 5 minutes and maximal effect in about 30 minutes (Figure 7.2). The effect of these agents generally wanes after 2 hours, and the often-stated 4-hour duration of action is somewhat optimistic. As a result, for regular use, these agents must be administered 4–6 times daily.

TABLE 7.2

Common β-agonist bronchodilator formulations

Drug	Metered-dose / dry powder inhaler (µg)	Nebulizer (mg [mg/mL])	Oral (mg)	Duration of action (h)
Fenoterol	100–200	0.5–2 [1]	–	4–6
Salbutamol (albuterol)	100, 200	2.5–5 [5]	2.5, 5	4–6
Terbutaline	400, 500	–	2.5, 5	4–6
Formoterol (eformoterol)	4.5–12	–	–	12+
Salmeterol	25–50	–	–	12+

Adapted from GOLD Workshop Report Executive Summary, April 2003 (www.goldcopd.com)

Currently, the most widely used agent is salbutamol, also known as albuterol (salbutamol is the recommended international non-proprietary name favored by the WHO, albuterol is the generic name in the USA). It is available in a number of formulations, including metered-dose inhaler formulations and nebulized solutions. Administration via a nebulizer may be appropriate for patients with extremely limited airflows or in individuals who cannot coordinate the use of a metered-dose inhaler. Many patients seem to derive benefit from the ritual aspects of applying the nebulizer mask. In some countries, patients prefer nebulizer therapy because it is covered to a greater degree by their healthcare insurance than are metered-dose inhaler formulations.

Side effects of β-agonists include ventricular contractions, palpitations, tachycardia, tremor, sleep disturbances and hypokalemia. These are systemic effects due to the total absorbed dose. While topical deposition in the airway by inhalation increases the therapeutic index, drug that is deposited in the mouth and swallowed can result in side effects without local benefit. Such side effects can be reduced by the use of spacers or other devices that decrease oral deposition of the drug.

Salbutamol is also available for oral use. As might be expected, for oral administration systemic dosing is considerably higher relative to the same lung dosing by inhalation. As a result, the side effects tachycardia and tremor are more common, so oral dosing is reserved for highly selected patients. Slow-release oral formulations of salbutamol permit its use as a long-acting preparation, but there is no change in the pharmacokinetics of the drug itself in these preparations.

Long-acting β-agonists. Two long-acting β-agonist bronchodilators are currently available: salmeterol and formoterol (eformoterol). Both are long-acting for pharmacokinetic reasons. Salmeterol interacts with two sites in the β-adrenergic receptor: the active site, to activate adenyl cyclase and thus cause cAMP production, and a second site that allows the drug to remain bound to the receptor and thus to have a long duration of action. The long duration of action of formoterol is probably due to its high lipophilicity; it binds to the cell membrane and remains there as a reservoir. Both drugs have a duration of action of 12 hours (Figure 7.2), making them appropriate for twice-daily dosing. The onset of action of formoterol is similar to that of salbutamol. Salmeterol has a much slower onset of action, requiring 15–30 minutes for bronchodilator effect and 2 hours for a maximal effect.

Anticholinergics affect cholinergic transmission, which is critical in maintaining normal airway smooth muscle tone. M_1 muscarinic receptors mediate neural transmission in the vagal ganglia, and M_3 muscarinic receptors at the neuromuscular junctions mediate smooth muscle contraction. Blockade of these receptors, particularly the M_3 receptors, can antagonize normal airway tone and thus result in bronchodilation. M_2 receptors have a feedback control function and may attenuate vagal activity.

Atropine has a modest bronchodilator effect, but is seldom used because of its other systemic effects. The anticholinergics most commonly used to achieve bronchodilation are quaternary amines (Table 7.3). When inhaled, these agents are absorbed very poorly, resulting in a high degree of local activity and a very low systemic side effect profile. Ipratropium bromide is most widely used. It has an onset of action slightly slower than salbutamol, with a bronchodilator effect in 10 minutes, a near-maximal effect in 30 minutes and a duration of action of 4–6 hours (Figure 7.2). It is available in a metered-dose inhaler and as a nebulized solution. The approved dose in most countries (42 μg or 2 puffs every 6 hours) is probably not at the top of the dose–response curve. As a result, improved bronchodilation and clinical effect can often be achieved with increased doses, and routine administration of 3 or 4 puffs has been suggested and is widely used. Interestingly, while the bronchodilator effect of ipratropium is clearly shorter than that of salmeterol, both drugs result in a similar degree of

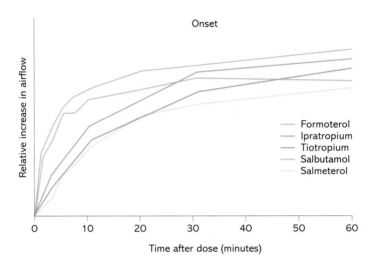

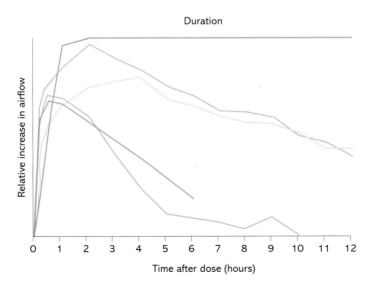

Figure 7.2 Onset and duration of action of bronchodilators.

improvement in exercise performance 6 hours following administration. This would be consistent with ipratropium improving lung volumes and reducing dynamic hyperinflation over and above its ability to improve airflow.

Tiotropium is a recently approved long-acting anticholinergic bronchodilator. It dissociates relatively rapidly from the M_2 muscarinic receptor, giving it some selectivity for the M_1 and M_3 receptors. Whether this is of clinical significance is unclear. Its long duration of action is due to its prolonged association with the M_1 and M_3 receptors. Its onset of action is slower than that of ipratropium, but the duration of action is noticeably longer (Figure 7.2). A bronchodilator effect is still detectable after 36 hours, and the maximal bronchodilator effect accumulates over the first few days of administration. Its duration of action makes it appropriate for use once a day.

Side effects from anticholinergics in clinical use are generally mild and include dry mouth and metallic taste. Closed-angle glaucoma may develop if drug is deposited in the eye. Men with prostate disease should be monitored for urinary tract effects, but these are uncommon. In asthmatics, paradoxical bronchoconstriction can occur.

TABLE 7.3

Amine anticholinergic bronchodilators

Drug	Metered-dose / dry powder inhaler (µg)	Nebulizer (mg)	Oral (mg)	Duration of action (h)
Atropine sulfate*	–	2.0	–	–
Ipratropium bromide	40–80	0.25–0.5	–	6–8
Oxitropium bromide	200	–	–	7–9
Tiotropium bromide	18	–	–	24–36

* The intravenous atropine preparation has been administered by nebulizer; it is not currently used, as it has adverse systemic effects

Theophylline is not effective topically as a bronchodilator and is usually used orally, though it can be administered rectally. It has several mechanisms of action, including inhibition of adenosine receptors and inhibition of multiple species of phosphodiesterase. The mechanism that leads to bronchodilation is unclear. The traditional concept of phosphodiesterase inhibition leading to increases in cAMP and bronchodilation has been called into question.

A number of theophylline preparations are available. Theophylline USP (United States Pharmacopeia) is comparatively inexpensive but has a relatively short duration of action. It is cleaved by hepatic enzymes, which are inducible by a variety of stimuli; this leads to marked variations in theophylline clearance between patients and even in a given patient with changes in clinical state. Slow-release theophylline preparations for use once or twice a day provide steadier blood levels and are easier to use clinically. However, theophylline has major adverse side effects, which limit its use. These include: central nervous system effects leading to nausea, vomiting and seizures; arrhythmias; relaxation of the lower gastroesophageal sphincter causing or worsening gastroesophageal reflux; diarrhea; and headaches. Drug–drug interactions are frequent and further complicate use in clinical practice.

Many clinicians routinely check theophylline blood levels, as toxic effects can be observed at levels only slightly above the traditional therapeutic range of 10–20 µg/mL. Recent practice, however, has been to use theophylline at relatively low doses, maintaining blood levels in the 5–10 µg/mL range. This range is often associated with a satisfying clinical response and has an increased safety margin. A further reason for repeated testing is that, as noted above, theophylline is metabolized by the liver, and hepatic clearance can change, resulting in varying blood levels despite constant dosing and good compliance.

Theophylline can also be combined with β-agonist bronchodilators (with which cAMP levels may be raised synergistically) and with ipratropium.

Combinations of bronchodilators from different classes are possible. While some studies have suggested that maximal bronchodilator effect can be achieved with a single agent given at sufficiently high dose, several large clinical trials have demonstrated improved bronchodilator effect when combinations of β-agonist and anticholinergic bronchodilators are administered. A commercially available combination of salbutamol and ipratropium (Combivent®) has achieved widespread clinical acceptance. Ipratropium can also be combined with long-acting β-agonist bronchodilators. Interestingly, when given together with salmeterol, ipratropium increases bronchodilation for considerably longer than the expected 4–6-hour duration. This is consistent with a synergistic interaction between these classes of bronchodilators.

Non-bronchodilator effects of bronchodilators. It is likely that all drugs used to achieve bronchodilation have a number of other effects. The clinical importance of these non-bronchodilator effects remains undefined.

Long-acting β-agonist bronchodilators and both long- and short-acting anticholinergic bronchodilators have been associated with a reduction in COPD exacerbation frequency in some studies. The mechanisms by which such an effect might be mediated are unclear. However, salmeterol has direct effects on airway epithelial cells that may mitigate epithelial damage secondary to bacterial infection. β-agonists may inhibit the activity of inflammatory cells and act on blood vessels to reduce the formation of and accelerate the clearance of edema.

Anticholinergics also have the potential for anti-inflammatory action by inhibiting the release of inflammatory mediators. The Lung Health Study assessed the ability of ipratropium to slow the rate at which lung function is lost in COPD; it was found to be without effect. Tiotropium has not been rigorously assessed in this regard.

Theophylline too may have anti-inflammatory actions in addition to its bronchodilator activity. It can improve diaphragmatic muscle contractility and may have other benefits, including a positive inotropic effect and a mild diuretic effect. In some studies, patients have reported subjective benefits from theophylline out of proportion to its modest bronchodilator activity.

Pharmacological treatment: corticosteroids

Oral glucocorticoids should be avoided if at all possible in the management of stable COPD (Table 7.4). Glucocorticoid-induced side effects are relatively common and can be devastating in COPD patients. Steroid myopathy may further compromise individuals already relatively unable to exercise. Steroid-induced osteoporosis may lead to fractures, which not only compromise mobility but also, if they occur in the spine or ribs, may lead to chest-wall splinting and an increased risk of pneumonia. Chronic administration of oral glucocorticoids has been associated with increased mortality in COPD patients. However, systemic glucocorticoids may be of benefit during COPD exacerbations (see below). Treatment should be stopped after 7–14 days.

Inhaled glucocorticoids have been evaluated in four large trials to determine whether they mitigate the rate of loss of lung function in COPD. All four studies failed to show a benefit. A recent meta-analysis, however, suggests that the available studies may have been underpowered and that a very small effect may be present. Nevertheless, inhaled glucocorticoids should not be used for this purpose, as current evidence does not show any benefit of these agents in the rate of decline in FEV_1.

Inhaled glucocorticoids may, however, improve airflow. The mechanisms underlying this effect are unclear, but reduction of airway edema has been suggested. It may take several weeks or even as much as 6 months for benefits of this treatment to be observed. Generally speaking, the improvement in airflow, if there is any, is much less than that achieved with bronchodilators, averaging about 50 mL compared with 200–300 mL achievable with bronchodilators (see above).

Inhaled glucocorticoids have also been reported to reduce exacerbation frequency and severity. This decrease appears to be associated with a beneficial effect on health status (quality of life), which is reasonable, as COPD exacerbations are associated with a worsening in health status. One large study demonstrated a statistically significant benefit in terms of both exacerbations and health status. The effect was driven primarily by the most severely affected patients (patients with an $FEV_1 < 1.25$ L) who experienced the most frequent

TABLE 7.4

Use of glucocorticoids in COPD

Systemic

- May be used short term (7–14 days) during exacerbations
- Avoid chronic use
- No rationale for a therapeutic challenge

Inhaled

- Modest bronchodilator effect
- Reduce exacerbation frequency/severity
- Improve health status
- No effect on rate of FEV_1 decline

exacerbations (> 2/year). Milder cases (FEV_1 > 1.5 L) with fewer exacerbations (1.2/year) did not benefit from inhaled glucocorticoids. Inhaled glucocorticoids should be therefore considered for patients experiencing frequent exacerbations, particularly if they are already receiving maximal bronchodilator therapy.

Combinations of inhaled glucocorticoids with long-acting β-agonist bronchodilators are available and approved for use in asthma. These agents have proved extremely popular. It is likely that there are collaborative and/or synergistic interactions between β-agonists and glucocorticoids which improve asthma control. Whether such benefits also accrue to the COPD patient remains to be determined.

Other pharmacological treatment

Vaccines. Influenza vaccination is recommended for all elderly patients since it can reduce their mortality from influenza by around 50%. It is particularly recommended for patients with COPD. The vaccine is adjusted each year to be effective against the appropriate strains, and the vaccination is given once in autumn or twice a year, in autumn and winter.

Streptococcus pneumonia is the commonest cause of community-acquired pneumonia, and pneumococcal infection is more common in adults over the age of 50. Pneumococcal vaccination has been shown to be beneficial in reducing mortality from *Streptococcus pneumonia* in an elderly population and, by extrapolation, might be expected to be effective in COPD patients. There are insufficient data to support its general use in COPD patients.

α_1-antitrypsin augmentation therapy. Patients with severe hereditary α_1-antitrypsin deficiency and established emphysema may be candidates for α_1-antitrypsin replacement therapy. Therapy is expensive and is not available in most countries, and rigorous controlled trials are still awaited. It is not recommended in patients with COPD that is unrelated to α_1-antitrypsin deficiency.

Antibiotics. Prophylactic, continuous use of antibiotics has not been shown to have any significant effect on frequent exacerbations of COPD. Thus, present evidence supports their use in treating the effects of exacerbations of COPD, but their long-term use is not recommended.

Mucolytic agents (ambroxol, carbocisteine, iodinated glycerol) have produced variable results in patients with COPD. Most studies have shown little or no change in lung function or symptoms. A systematic Cochrane collaborative review showed that they reduce episodes of acute-on-chronic bronchitis compared with placebo. Their use, however, still remains controversial.

The mucolytic and antioxidant drug N-acetylcysteine has been shown to reduce the frequency of exacerbations of COPD.

Antitussives. Cough is a troublesome symptom in COPD, but it does have a protective role and therefore the use of antitussives is contraindicated in stable COPD.

Vasodilators. The rationale for the use of vasodilators is based on the relationship between pulmonary arterial pressure and mortality in COPD. Numerous vasodilators have been assessed. Most produce small changes in pulmonary arterial pressure, but at the expense of worsening ventilation–perfusion mismatching and therefore worsening gas exchange. There is therefore no indication for vasodilators in COPD.

Other drugs, such as leukotriene antagonists and nedocromil, have not been assessed in COPD and cannot be recommended.

Non-pharmacological treatment

Rehabilitation. Previously, the main management goals in COPD were prevention of deterioration of the condition, principally by encouraging smoking cessation, and improvement of lung function and thus symptoms with bronchodilators. There is now substantial evidence that improving quality of life, or health status, and the functional ability of patients is another attainable goal. The fact that the airflow limitation in COPD is largely irreversible means that the results of pharmacological therapy on lung function are at best modest. It is now known that, without changing airflow limitation, pulmonary rehabilitation can still improve performance status and health status.

The principal goals of pulmonary rehabilitation are reduced symptoms, improved health status and increased physical and emotional participation in everyday activities. These goals are particularly relevant in the moderate to severe stages of COPD, when breathlessness may result in the avoidance of activity. This results in deconditioning of the skeletal muscles, which in turn leads to increasing disability, social isolation and depression. This compounds the problems of dyspnea and lack of fitness, and a vicious circle ensues, resulting in increasing dependence and disability and worsening quality of life (Figure 7.3). The aim of pulmonary rehabilitation is to break this vicious circle of increasing inactivity, breathlessness and physical deconditioning, and improve exercise capacity and functional status.

The main components of a pulmonary rehabilitation program are:
• exercise training
• nutritional counseling
• education.

At all stages of the disease, patients with COPD appear to benefit from exercise training programs which improve exercise tolerance, symptoms of breathlessness and fatigue. Pulmonary rehabilitation has been assessed in numerous large clinical trials and the benefits are summarized in Table 7.5. Studies suggest that these benefits can be sustained after a single rehabilitation program if the patient maintains the exercise training at home.

The social isolation that accompanies severe COPD can lead to mood disturbances, which may require treatment. Encouragement of social contact is important, and contact in the rehabilitation group may provide support. Generally, rehabilitation programs consist of two or three sessions per week for 6–8 weeks and provide a program of exercises which the patient also performs between sessions. The improvement seen with pulmonary rehabilitation programs seems to be long-lasting, persisting for at least a year. Follow-up is beneficial, and occasional repeat sessions have been offered in some centers that provide continuing support.

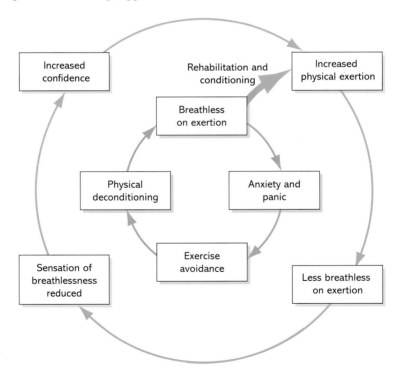

Figure 7.3 The vicious cycle of deconditioning and inactivity that occurs in COPD, and the effect of pulmonary rehabilitation.

Rehabilitation involves a multidisciplinary group of healthcare professionals, and the benefits from rehabilitation have been reported in inpatient, outpatient and home settings. Selection criteria for pulmonary rehabilitation programs are still under investigation. However, benefits are seen in patients over a wide range of disability, although those who are very severely disabled, for example those who are chairbound or have an MRC dyspnea grade of 5, may not derive any benefit.

It is important that motivated patients are selected for pulmonary rehabilitation programs. While many believe that inclusion of patients in a pulmonary rehabilitation program should be conditional on their participation in a smoking cessation program, there is no evidence that smokers will benefit less than non-smokers.

Exercise training to recondition skeletal muscles and improve exercise endurance is a key component of pulmonary rehabilitation. Bicycle ergometry and treadmill exercise are both suitable aerobic activities. A number of physiological variables, such as maximum oxygen consumption, maximum heart rate and maximum work performed are measured. A less complex approach utilizes a self-paced walking test, for example a 6-minute walking distance. Shuttle walking tests reflect an individual's peak oxygen consumption fairly accurately,

TABLE 7.5

Benefits of pulmonary rehabilitation in COPD

- Improves exercise capacity
- Reduces the perceived intensity of breathlessness
- Can improve health-related quality of life
- Reduces the number of hospitalizations and length of hospital stay
- Strength and endurance training of the upper limbs improves arm function
- Benefits extend well beyond the immediate period of training
- Improves survival
- Respiratory muscle training is beneficial, especially when combined with general exercise training
- Psychosocial intervention is helpful

provide more information than a 6-minute walking distance and are simpler to perform than a treadmill test.

Exercise training is performed regularly in a form that the patient will be able to continue at home during and after the rehabilitation program. The frequency of exercise varies from daily to weekly, the duration from 10 to 45 minutes and the intensity from 50% of peak oxygen consumption to maximum tolerated. The optimum length of a rehabilitation program has not been determined, and suggestions from randomized controlled trials vary between 4 and 10 weeks.

Some programs include training of specific muscle groups such as upper limb girdle muscles and aim to improve the patient's performance of specific tasks associated with daily living. There are no randomized controlled trial data to support the routine use of these exercises, but they may be useful in patients with comorbidity that restricts other forms of exercise or in those with severe COPD who find aerobic exercise too demanding.

The role of respiratory muscle training in pulmonary rehabilitation is still controversial. Training respiratory muscles for both strength and endurance has produced equivocal results in patients with COPD.

Nutritional counseling is based on the fact that the nutritional status of patients with COPD has an important effect on symptoms, disability and prognosis. Being overweight or underweight can be problematic. Around 25% of patients with moderate to severe COPD have a reduction in both their body mass index and fat-free mass index. Low body mass index has been shown to be an independent risk factor for mortality in COPD patients (see Figure 2.4).

The cause of malnutrition in COPD is complex and may relate to raised levels of various cytokines, including tumor necrosis factor. Reduced calorie intake can result when patients become breathless while eating. These patients should be encouraged to take small, frequent meals. Any problems with dentition should be corrected, and any comorbidity that might result in weight loss should be dealt with. Nutritional support in the form of increased calorie intake is best accompanied by exercise regimens that have an anabolic action. Underweight COPD patients whose nutritional state improves in response to therapy may improve respiratory muscle strength and have better survival statistics.

Obese patients with COPD are more likely to have greater impairment of activity and a greater degree of breathlessness than patients of normal weight. These patients should be encouraged to lose weight while taking regular exercise.

Education is included in most pulmonary rehabilitation programs, although its effect is unclear. Smoking cessation is a critical part of pulmonary rehabilitation and may be facilitated by advice and support from the physician. Advice should also be given on drug treatment and how to manage exacerbations.

Oxygen therapy. Long-term administration of oxygen therapy ($\geq$ 15 h/day) has been shown to:

- improve survival
- prevent progression of pulmonary hypertension
- decrease polycythemia.

The UK MRC trial of oxygen, 15 h/day, showed an increase in 5-year survival from 25% to 41% (compared with no oxygen), and a further trial, the Nocturnal Oxygen Therapy Trial (NOTT), showed that continuous oxygen therapy with a mean use of 17.7 h/day was more beneficial in terms of survival than use for only 12 h/day, which conferred no benefit. It is debatable whether oxygen therapy improves health status, but both mood and indices of depression improve.

Oxygen therapy reduces the oxygen costs of breathing and minute ventilation, thus reducing the sensation of breathlessness. It has been given to control severe breathlessness on exercise. Recent data suggest that ambulatory oxygen therapy improves the benefits obtained from exercise training programs.

When given during exercise, oxygen therapy increases walking distance by optimizing oxygen uptake and utilization by the muscles. However, there are no data indicating that long-term continuous oxygen therapy improves exercise capacity. Oxygen is administered during exercise to patients who usually fit the criteria for long-term oxygen therapy or to those who experience significant oxygen desaturation during exercise.

The goal of oxygen therapy is to increase the PaO_2 to at least 8 kPa (60 mmHg) or to produce an oxygen saturation (SaO_2) of at least 90% to ensure adequate oxygen delivery to vital organs. The treatment should be given to patients who have severe COPD with a PaO_2 below 7.3 kPa (55 mmHg) and an SaO_2 below 88%, with or without hypercapnia, or those with a PaO_2 between 7.3 and 8 kPa (55 and 60 mmHg) or an SaO_2 of 89% with evidence of pulmonary hypertension or peripheral edema and polycythemia (hematocrit over 55%). It should be assessed when the patient is in a clinically stable state, at least 6 weeks from the last exacerbation and when other drug therapy has been optimized.

Long-term oxygen therapy is usually provided in the form of an oxygen concentrator via nasal prongs with a flow rate of 2–3 L/minute. Patients who desaturate during exercise are often told to increase the flow rate during exercise. Portable oxygen can be provided by liquid oxygen and a portable device or by lightweight oxygen cylinders.

Oxygenation in air travel may be insufficient for patients with severe COPD, who should in any case seek advice about any form of travel. Modern aircraft cabin pressures have oxygen levels equivalent to those 1500–2500 m (5000–8000 feet) above sea level, that is, ambient oxygen pressures of 15–18 kPa (112–135 mmHg). This means that in a healthy individual the PaO_2 will reduce from 12 to 8.7 kPa (90 to 65 mmHg) and the SaO_2 from 96% to 90%. This degree of reduction in oxygenation may be hazardous in a patient with severe lung disease and hypoxia unless supplementary oxygen is given during the flight. Patients with COPD are considered able to fly safely, with supplementary oxygen, if:

- FEV_1 > 25% of the predicted value
- PaO_2 during flight > 6.7 kPa (50 mmHg)

Patients with a resting PaO_2 at sea level of > 9.3 kPa (70 mmHg) may safely fly without supplementary oxygen.

If there is any doubt about the advisability of air travel, patients can be referred for assessment to a respiratory physician, who may perform a hypoxic challenge, in which the patient breathes air with reduced levels of oxygen to assess their likely response to the levels of oxygen present during air travel.

Ventilatory support. The success of non-invasive intermittent positive-pressure ventilation (NIPPV) in patients with respiratory failure in exacerbations of COPD has led to its application to patients with chronic respiratory failure due to severe COPD. Several studies have examined the use of ventilatory support in such patients but have found no convincing evidence that this treatment produces a long-term survival advantage over oxygen therapy alone. Given the conflicting evidence for the use of long-term NIPPV, it cannot be recommended for the routine treatment of patients with chronic respiratory failure due to COPD. However, a combination of NIPPV with long-term oxygen therapy may help in some patients with severe daytime hypercapnia.

Surgical treatment of COPD

Bullectomy. Some patients with COPD develop large cyst-like spaces, or bullae, in the lungs, which tend to compress the more normal areas of the lung. Removal of bullae that do not contribute to gas exchange may allow decompression of the adjacent lung parenchyma. Bullae can be detected on plain chest radiographs, but are better viewed on CT scans, which also permit the assessment of emphysema in the remaining lung. This may be an important determinant of success in bullectomy.

A range of surgical procedures has been used, including bronchoscopic techniques using laser ablation. In carefully selected patients, such a procedure can improve lung function and symptoms of breathlessness. Patients who would benefit are those who have normal or minimally reduced DLCO and those who are not hypoxemic and who have good perfusion in the remaining lung, as assessed by lung perfusion scanning. Individuals less likely to benefit are those with pulmonary hypertension, hypercapnia and severe emphysema in the remaining non-bullous lung.

Lung volume reduction surgery (LVRS) removes emphysematous parts of the lung to decrease overinflation, thus improving the mechanical efficiency of the respiratory muscles, particularly the diaphragm. LVRS also increases the elastic recoil pressure of the lung, so improving expiratory flow rates. This operation can be performed unilaterally or

Key points – therapy in stable disease

- Bronchodilators are first-line treatment in COPD.
- Bronchodilators of various classes can be effectively used concurrently.
- Bronchodilators may have beneficial non-bronchodilator effects.
- Inhaled glucocorticoids can improve airflow modestly and can reduce exacerbation frequency and severity.
- Inhaled glucocorticoids do not slow the loss of lung function.
- Short courses (7–14 days) of systemic glucocorticoids may help following exacerbations but should not be used over the long term.
- Modest improvements in FEV_1 measured at rest may be associated with satisfying clinical responses, particularly on exertion.
- Optimum clinical benefits require an integrated program combining rehabilitation with pharmacotherapy.
- Influenza vaccination is recommended for patients with COPD.
- There is some support for pneumococcal vaccination in COPD.
- Long-term oxygen therapy improves survival in patients with hypoxemic COPD.
- Long-term oxygen therapy is required ≥ 15 h/day to be effective.
- Ambulatory oxygen may be beneficial in some patients.
- Surgical removal of large bullae may improve lung function and symptoms in selected cases.
- Lung volume reduction surgery may be of benefit with careful patient selection.
- Lung transplantations are usually performed on patients below the age of 50 years.
- Body mass index (BMI) has been shown to be an important predictor of survival in patients with COPD.
- Patients with low BMI who can increase their weight show improved survival.
- Rehabilitation has been shown to be beneficial in terms of improving exercise tolerance, symptoms of breathlessness and fatigue in patients with COPD.

bilaterally using mediastinotomy or video-assisted thoracoscopy, and in good centers mortality is under 5%.

Selection criteria for those who would derive most benefit are not fully established, although most studies select patients with an FEV_1 < 35% predicted, a PaO_2 < 6 kPa (45 mmHg), predominant upper-lobe emphysema on the CT scan and a residual volume of > 200% predicted. Studies have shown that very severely affected patients with homogeneous disease and FEV_1 or DLCO < 25% predicted do not benefit; indeed, there is an increased mortality in this group. Conversely, the US National Emphysema Treatment Trial identified individuals with upper-lobe disease and exercise limitation despite optimal medical treatment and rehabilitation as a group of good responders. LVRS has been shown to improve FEV_1, decrease total lung capacity and improve exercise tolerance and quality of life; these effects may last for more than 2 years.

Lung transplantation. In patients with very advanced COPD, lung transplantation has been shown to improve health status and functional capacity, although it does not convey a survival benefit. The main criteria for lung transplantation are FEV_1 < 35% of predicted, PaO_2 < 7.3–8.0 kPa (55–60 mmHg), $PaCO_2$ > 6.7 kPa (50 mmHg) and secondary pulmonary hypertension; patients should be under 50 years of age. The number of lung transplants is limited by a shortage of donors. Complications in patients with COPD after transplantation include rejection, bronchiolitis obliterans and opportunistic infection. Bronchiolitis occurs in 30% of patients surviving for 5 years and may be fatal. Patients require long-term immunosuppressive therapy.

Key references

Aalbers R et al. Formoterol in patients with chronic obstructive pulmonary disease: a randomized, controlled, 3-month trial. *Eur Respir J* 2002;19:936–43.

British Thoracic Society Standards of Care Committee. Managing passengers with respiratory disease planning air travel. *Thorax* 2002;57:289–304.

Calverley P, Pauwels R, Vestbo J et al. Combined salmeterol and fluticasone in the treatment of chronic obstructive pulmonary disease: a randomised controlled trial. *Lancet* 2003;361:449–56.

Casaburi R, Mahler DA, Jones PW et al. A long-term evaluation of once-daily inhaled tiotropium in chronic obstructive pulmonary disease. *Eur Respir J* 2002;19:217–24.

COMBIVENT Inhalation Solution Study Group. Routine nebulized ipratropium and albuterol together are better than either alone in COPD. *Chest* 1997;112:1514–21.

Cooper CB. Domiciliary oxygen therapy. In: Calverley PMA, Pride NB, eds. *Chronic Obstructive Pulmonary Disease*. London: Chapman & Hall, 1995:495–526.

Global Initiative for Chronic Obstructive Lung Disease. *Global Strategy for the Diagnosis, Management, and Prevention of Chronic Obstructive Pulmonary Disease. NHLBI/WHO Workshop Report*. National Heart, Lung, and Blood Institute (USA), World Health Organization: 2001, updated 2003. www.goldcopd.com

Griffiths TL, Phillips CJ, Davies S et al. Cost-effectiveness of an outpatient multidisciplinary pulmonary rehabilitation programme. *Thorax* 2001;56:779–784.

Johnson M, Rennard SI. Alternative mechanisms for long-acting beta$_2$-adrenergic agonists in COPD. *Chest* 2001;120:258–70.

Lacasse Y, Wong E, Guyatt GH et al. Meta-analysis of respiratory rehabilitation in chronic obstructive pulmonary disease. *Lancet* 1996;348:1115–19.

Medical Research Council Oxygen Working Party Report. Long-term domiciliary oxygen therapy in chronic carboxy cor pulmonale complicating chronic bronchitis and emphysema. *Lancet* 1981;1:681–6.

Morgan M, Singh S. *Practical Pulmonary Rehabilitation*. London: Chapman & Hall Medical, 1997.

National Emphysema Treatment Trial Research Group. A randomized trial comparing lung-volume–reduction surgery with medical therapy for severe emphysema. *N Engl J Med* 2003;348:2058–73.

Nocturnal Oxygen Therapy Trial Group. Continuous or nocturnal oxygen therapy in hypoxic chronic obstructive lung disease. *Ann Int Med* 1980;93:391–8.

O'Brien GM, Griner GJ. Surgery for severe COPD. Lung volume reduction and lung transplantation. *Postgrad Med J* 1998;103:179–94.

Paggiaro PL, Dahle R, Bakran I et al. Multicentre randomised placebo-controlled trial of inhaled fluticasone propionate in patients with chronic obstructive pulmonary disease. International COPD Study Group. *Lancet* 1998;351:773–80.

Pauwels R, Buist AS, Calverley PM et al. The GOLD Scientific Committee. Global strategy for the diagnosis, management, and prevention of chronic obstructive pulmonary disease. NHLBI/WHO Global Initiative for Chronic Obstructive Lung Disease (GOLD) Workshop summary. *Am J Respir Crit Care Med* 2001;163:1256–76.

Rennard SI, Serby CW, Ghafouri M et al. Extended therapy with ipratropium is associated with improved lung function in COPD: A retrospective analysis of data from seven clinical trials. *Chest* 1996;110:62–70.

Rennard SI, Anderson W, ZuWallack R et al. Use of a long-acting inhaled beta$_2$-adrenergic agonist, salmeterol xinafoate, in patients with chronic obstructive pulmonary disease. *Am J Respir Crit Care Med* 2001;163:1087–9.

Rennard SI. Anticholinergics in combination bronchodilator therapy in COPD. In: Spector SL, ed. *Anticholinergic Agents in the Upper and Lower Airways*. New York: Marcel Dekker, 1999:119–36.

Royal College of Physicians of London Domiciliary Oxygen Therapy Services. *Clinical Guidelines and Advice for Prescribers*. London: Royal College of Physicians, 1999.

Schols AMWJ, Slangen J, Volovics L, Wouters EF. Weight loss is a reversible factor in the prognosis of chronic obstructive pulmonary disease. *Am J Respir Crit Care Med* 1998;157:1791–7.

Szafranski W, Cukier A, Ramirez A et al. Efficacy and safety of budesonide/formoterol in the management of chronic obstructive pulmonary disease. *Eur Respir J* 2003;21:74–81.

van Noord JA, de Munck DRAJ, Bantje TA et al. Long-term treatment of chronic obstructive pulmonary disease with salmeterol and the additive effect of ipratropium. *Eur Respir J* 2000;15:878–85.

Vincken W, van Noord JA, Greefhorst AP et al. Improved health outcomes in patients with COPD during 1 year's treatment with tiotropium. *Eur Respir J* 2002;19: 209–16.

Acute exacerbations of COPD place a large burden on healthcare resources. It has been estimated that in an average UK Health Authority with a population of 250 000, there will be 14 200 consultations with a family physician and 680 hospital admissions for exacerbations of COPD per year. In the UK, respiratory admissions account for 25% of all acute emergency admissions, and COPD accounts for more than half of these, representing 203 193 hospital admissions in 1994. A UK survey of medical admissions found that 73% of male and 23% of female respiratory admissions in the age range 65–74 years were due to COPD. Recent studies have suggested that up to 50% of patients do not report exacerbations, so the true frequency is much higher than the number of consultations with family physicians suggests. Thus, the healthcare burden imposed by exacerbations of COPD is enormous.

Definition

There is currently no general agreement on the definition of an exacerbation of COPD. Most definitions of exacerbations are based on increasing symptoms and/or increased healthcare utilization. A commonly used definition is based on the type and number of symptoms, such as increases in dyspnea, sputum volume or sputum purulence with or without symptoms of upper respiratory infection, and is subdivided into type I, II and III depending on the number of symptoms (Table 8.1). Most studies have defined exacerbations as worsening of symptoms requiring changes in normal treatment, including increased bronchodilator therapy, use of antimicrobial therapy or use of short courses of oral corticosteroids. The severity of an exacerbation can also be defined in terms of increasing healthcare utilization as: mild (self-managed by the patients at home); moderate (requiring treatment by the family physician and/or hospital outpatient attendance); or severe (resulting in admission to hospital). The severity of an exacerbation and the consequent healthcare utilization may depend on the severity of the underlying COPD. Recently an

TABLE 8.1

Definition of COPD exacerbation

Type I

Three of: increased breathlessness, sputum volume or sputum purulence

Type II

Two of: increased breathlessness, sputum volume or sputum purulence

Type III

One of: increased breathlessness, sputum volume or sputum purulence

plus

one of the following symptoms:

- upper respiratory infection (sore throat, nasal discharge) within the past 5 days
- fever without other cause
- increased wheezing
- increased cough
- increase in respiratory or heart rate by 20% compared with baseline

Source: Anthonisen et al. 1987

exacerbation of COPD has been defined as 'a sustained worsening of the patient's condition from the stable state and beyond normal day-to-day variations that is acute in onset and necessitates a change in medication in a patient with underlying COPD'. Sustained worsening is defined as symptoms worse than normal for at least 24 hours. A staging system for exacerbations of COPD has recently been proposed using clinical descriptors to characterize acute exacerbations (Table 8.2).

Pathology

Studies of the pathology of exacerbations of COPD have been performed in postmortem material and bronchial biopsies. Recently, inflammation has also been assessed by non-invasive surrogate markers in sputum and breath. Relatively few of these last studies have involved patients with COPD, and patient numbers have been small.

TABLE 8.2

Staging of COPD exacerbations based on healthcare utilization

Severity	Level of healthcare utilization
Mild	Patients have an increased need for medication, which they can manage in their own normal environment
Moderate	Patients have an increased need for medication and feel the need to seek additional medical assistance
Severe	Patients/caregivers recognize obvious and/or rapid deterioration in condition, requiring hospitalization

It has been assumed that increased inflammation in the airways is a characteristic feature of exacerbations of COPD. However, the presence of increased inflammation and particularly the type of inflammation that is present is controversial and depends on whether the inflammatory response is assessed in sputum, bronchoalveolar lavage fluid or bronchial biopsy, and on the severity of the exacerbation. The few studies of biopsies from patients with exacerbations of COPD have been in patients with predominantly chronic bronchitis with mild airflow limitation; in some of these studies, increased levels of eosinophils are present in induced sputum and in bronchial biopsies from patients with exacerbations. However, neutrophils are also present in increased numbers in the bronchial walls and in bronchoalveolar lavage fluid in exacerbations of COPD.

Surrogate markers of inflammation, such as sputum levels of tumor necrosis factor α, IL-8 and IL-6, have been shown to be elevated in exacerbations of COPD. Oxidative stress is a major component of the airway inflammation in COPD, and surrogate markers of oxidative stress are known to be elevated in blood, exhaled breath and breath condensate in stable COPD compared with levels in healthy smokers, with further increases measured during exacerbations of COPD.

Etiology

The main etiologic factors in exacerbations of COPD are thought to be bacterial and viral infections and air pollutants. Other factors associated with exacerbations of COPD are social deprivation and changes in temperature. However, in around 30% of exacerbations of COPD no obvious etiologic factor is found.

Bacteria. Between 30% and 50% of patients with exacerbations of COPD have a positive sputum culture for bacteria. However, around 20–30% of clinically stable patients also have a positive bacterial culture from sputum. Bronchoscopic protected specimen brush biopsies show that bacteria are present in the lower airways in greater numbers during exacerbations than in the stable clinical state, suggesting infection. The main organisms present in sputum in exacerbations of COPD are *Haemophilus influenzae*, *Streptococcus pneumoniae* and *Moraxella catarrhalis*. Gram-negative bacteria such as *Pseudomonas aeruginosa* are less common during exacerbations of COPD, but occur with increasing frequency in patients with severe airflow limitation. In some studies, atypical bacterial pathogens such as *Chlamydia pneumoniae* have been found during exacerbations of COPD. Changes in bacterial strain have also been associated with acute exacerbation.

Respiratory viruses. Several studies have shown that viruses are present in around 30% of acute exacerbations of COPD. They are associated with increased inflammation in the airways and a more prolonged time to the resolution of symptoms.

Air pollution is now well established as a cause of exacerbations of COPD. Epidemiological studies show links between the levels of particulate air pollution and emergency admissions for exacerbations of COPD. Other air pollutants, such as ozone, have also been associated with exacerbations of COPD in epidemiological studies.

Natural history
Studies in the 1960s, particularly in the UK, suggested that exacerbations of COPD were associated with small and transient decreases in respiratory function, and therefore did not alter the natural history of the disease. However, this view has recently been challenged, and it is believed there may be an accelerated decline in lung function

as a result of exacerbations of COPD. There are several large population studies showing that the number of exacerbations experienced correlates with the severity of the underlying disease. The median number of exacerbations in patients with severe COPD is around 2.2–2.5 exacerbations per year.

Follow-up of patients with exacerbations of COPD shows a high readmission rate of around 30% over the first 3 months. Patients with recurrent exacerbations (three or more exacerbations per year) have a higher mortality and decreased quality of life.

Prevention

Prevention or reduction of the severity or length of exacerbations of COPD is a major goal in the management of COPD. Influenza vaccination is recommended since it reduces hospitalization for pneumonia in elderly patients with COPD during epidemic periods. Vaccination against *Streptococcus* pneumonia is available and is effective in preventing infective complications of streptococcal pneumonia. However, the value of the vaccination specifically for COPD patients is still debated.

There is now evidence that inhaled corticosteroids may prevent exacerbations of COPD and reduce their severity. High-dose inhaled corticosteroids (fluticasone, 1 mg/day) reduced exacerbation rates by 25% (from 1.32/year with placebo to 0.99/year with inhaled corticosteroids). In this study, the health status of patients receiving inhaled corticosteroids deteriorated at a significantly slower rate than did that of those receiving placebo. The positive effect of inhaled corticosteroids may result from their influence on exacerbations of COPD. This effect is seen only in patients with moderate to severe COPD. At present, the recommendation is that inhaled corticosteroids might reduce exacerbations in those with FEV_1 less than 50% of predicted and two or more exacerbations per year.

Other drugs have also been shown to prevent or reduce exacerbation rates. A meta-analysis of randomized controlled trials of the antioxidant/mucolytic drug N-acetylcysteine showed that it was of value in reducing the frequency of exacerbations of COPD; long-acting anticholinergic and β-agonist bronchodilators may also do so.

Symptoms and signs

Patients with acute exacerbations typically present with increased cough, changes in sputum volume and/or purulence, and increased breathlessness, wheezing and chest tightness. Clinical history, examination and arterial blood gases are used to assess the severity of exacerbations in order to judge whether patients require admission to hospital.

Respiratory failure may or may not be present, as may cyanosis and the flapping tremor of hypercapnia, but these signs are rather insensitive. Pulse oximetry can provide rapid information on oxygen saturation, but arterial blood gases should be measured in all patients with severe exacerbations. PEF measurements are not as useful for determining the need for hospital admission in COPD as they are in asthma.

Management

The aims of management in exacerbations of COPD are to relieve airway obstruction, correct hypoxemia, address any comorbid disorder that may contribute to respiratory deterioration and treat any precipitating causes such as infection.

Management at home. Most exacerbations of COPD are treated in primary care; a minority of patients are admitted to hospital. Criteria have been suggested to determine which patients may be more suitable for hospital admission; however, these guidelines have not been fully tested (Table 8.3).

Bronchodilator dose and frequency are increased in home management of exacerbations of COPD. If not already used, therapy with multiple bronchodilator classes may be added if symptoms are not improving. In the most severe cases, high-dose nebulized bronchodilators can be given on a regular or as-required basis for several days. However, there is evidence that the use of multiple doses of bronchodilators by metered-dose inhaler with a spacer device has an effect similar to that of nebulized bronchodilators in exacerbations of COPD. When a nebulizer is used, it is probably safer to use air as the driving gas, rather than oxygen, and to continue oxygen by nasal

TABLE 8.3

Indications for hospital admission for acute exacerbations of COPD

The more referral indicators that are present, the more likely the need for admission to hospital

	Treat at home	Treat in hospital
Ability to cope at home	Yes	No
Breathlessness	Mild	Severe
General condition	Good	Poor – deteriorating
Level of activity	Good	Poor / confined to bed
Cyanosis	No	Yes
Worsening peripheral edema	No	Yes
Level of consciousness	Normal	Impaired
Already receiving long-term oxygen therapy	No	Yes
Social circumstances	Good	Living alone / not coping
Acute confusion	No	Yes
Rapid rate of onset	No	Yes
Changes on the chest radiograph	No	Present
Arterial pH level	≥ 7.35	< 7.35
PaO_2	≥ 7 kPa (52 mmHg)	< 7 kPa (52 mmHg)

PaO_2, partial pressure of oxygen in arterial blood
Source: British Thoracic Society Guidelines for the management of chronic obstructive pulmonary disease. *Thorax* 1997;52 (suppl 5):S1–S28.

prongs. The long-term use of nebulized therapy after acute exacerbations of COPD is not routinely recommended.

Antibiotic use in exacerbations of COPD is still controversial. In mild to moderate exacerbations, sputum culture is not usually necessary. Patients with two or more of the symptoms of increased breathlessness, sputum production and sputum purulence show greater improvement with antibiotics than with placebo during exacerbations of COPD. Simple antibiotics, modified according to local bacterial resistance patterns, should be used. Amoxicillin can be given in most cases as the first-line treatment, or co-amoxiclav in those who fail to respond or who are known or suspected to have β-lactamase-producing organisms in their sputum. Clarithromycin is an alternative in patients who are hypersensitive to penicillins.

Corticosteroid use in exacerbations in COPD is now well established. Four controlled trials have shown that systemic corticosteroids achieve a greater improvement in spirometry, reduced length of stay in hospital and decreased treatment failure than placebo. The exact dose of corticosteroids that should be given in exacerbations of COPD has not yet been established, but on present evidence 30 mg/day for 10 days is appropriate.

Hospital treatment. Provisional guidelines suggest indications for hospital admission for acute exacerbations of COPD (Table 8.3). Blood gases should be measured in all severe exacerbations of COPD. A PaO_2 < 6.7 kPa (50 mmHg), a $PaCO_2$ > 9.3 kPa (70 mmHg) or a pH < 7.3 suggests a life-threatening episode that needs close monitoring or intensive care unit (ICU) management.

The presence of a pulmonary embolism, which can mimic the clinical syndrome of an exacerbation of COPD, can be very difficult to diagnose, particularly in COPD. Chest radiographs are useful in identifying this alternative diagnosis. A low diastolic blood pressure and an inability to increase PaO_2 to > 8 kPa (60 mmHg) despite oxygen therapy also suggest pulmonary embolism. Spiral CT pulmonary angiography is the best tool available for the diagnosis of pulmonary embolism. Ventilation/perfusion scanning is of no value in patients with COPD.

The first actions in treating hospitalized patients with an exacerbation of COPD are to provide controlled oxygen therapy and to determine whether the exacerbation is life-threatening, in which case admission to high-dependency unit (HDU) or ICU is indicated. Management of other acute exacerbations of COPD is summarized in Table 8.4.

Oxygen therapy aims to maintain adequate oxygenation

(PaO_2 > 8 kPa (60 mmHg) or saturation > 90%) without worsening

TABLE 8.4

Management of severe but not life-threatening exacerbations of COPD

- Assess severity of symptoms, blood gases, chest radiograph
- Administer controlled oxygen therapy – repeat arterial blood gas measurement after 30 minutes
- Bronchodilators
  - increase dose or frequency
  - combine β-agonists and anticholinergics
  - use spacers or air-driven nebulizers
  - consider adding intravenous aminophylline, if needed
- Glucocorticosteroids, oral or intravenous
- Antibiotics when signs of bacterial infection are present, oral or occasionally intravenous
- Consider mechanical ventilation
- At all times:
  - monitor fluid balance and nutrition
  - consider subcutaneous heparin
  - identify and treat associated conditions (e.g. heart failure, arrhythmias)
  - closely monitor condition of the patient

hypercapnia. Many patients who have chronic hypoxemia will tolerate lower levels of oxygen (PaO_2 > 6.7 kPa, 50 mmHg) after administration of oxygen. Oxygen is given in inspired concentrations of 24–28% oxygen by Venturi mask or 1–2 liters/minute by nasal prongs. Arterial blood gases should be measured to ensure satisfactory oxygenation without additional CO_2 retention and consequent acidosis. Oxygen masks provide a more accurate inspired oxygen concentration, but nasal prongs are better tolerated.

Bronchodilator therapy can mitigate the effects of increased airway obstruction in patients with exacerbations of COPD, namely increased respiratory work of breathing – hyperinflation, respiratory muscle mechanical disadvantage and impaired ventilation/perfusion matching, causing hypoxemia. Short-acting β-agonists are preferred as initial bronchodilators for the treatment of acute exacerbations of COPD. Although they are usually given in nebulized form, there is evidence that administration of β-agonists via metered-dose inhaler and spacer device is equally efficacious. Nebulizers should be powered by compressed air rather than oxygen if $PaCO_2$ is raised, to prevent worsening hypercapnia and acidosis. Oxygen administration by nasal prongs can continue at 1–2 liters/minute during nebulization. If the response to β-agonist drugs is not prompt, or if the patient has a very severe exacerbation, the anticholinergic drug ipratropium bromide can be added.

The role of intravenous aminophylline in the treatment of exacerbations of COPD is controversial. Studies have shown minor improvements in lung volumes following administration of aminophylline, but also worsening gas exchange. Monitoring the serum theophylline is recommended to avoid side effects of these drugs.

Glucocorticoids have been shown in several studies to be effective in reducing symptoms and improving lung function in patients with acute exacerbations of COPD. Currently, systemic corticosteroids, 30 mg/day for 10 days, are recommended for all patients with acute exacerbations in the absence of significant contraindications. Corticosteroids should be discontinued after the acute episode; clinical improvement with corticosteroids during the exacerbation does not necessarily indicate the need for long-term oral or inhaled corticosteroids.

Antibiotic therapy in exacerbations of COPD was the subject of a meta-analysis of nine randomized, placebo-controlled trials. This analysis established a small but significant benefit, which was most evident in patients with the most symptoms. When two of the three cardinal symptoms (increasing breathlessness, increasing sputum volume and increasing sputum purulence) were present, there was a significant improvement with antibiotics over placebo.

In most cases, sputum Gram stain or culture is not necessary. Oral rather than intravenous antibiotics should be given. Failure to respond to simple antibiotics (as described above), the known presence of β-lactamase-producing organisms in sputum, or severe exacerbations all suggest the use of antibiotics with a broader spectrum such as co-amoxiclav or a second- or third-generation cephalosporin or fluoroquinolone or newer macrolide.

The hypothesis that recurrent bacterial infections have a role in the progression of COPD remains unproven.

Sputum clearance. Airway inflammation in exacerbations of COPD promotes mucus hypersecretion. There are no convincing data to support the use of pharmacological agents to improve mucokinetics during exacerbations. The use of mechanical techniques such as physiotherapy have no proven value in acute exacerbations of COPD, unless a large amount of sputum (> 25 mL) is produced daily or there is mucus plugging with lobar atelectasis. Physiotherapy is not recommended in patients with acute-on-chronic respiratory failure.

Diuretics are indicated in the presence of edema and raised jugular venous pressure.

Anticoagulants, specifically prophylactic subcutaneous heparin, should be administered to patients with severe exacerbations of COPD, particularly those who are immobile and those with acute-on-chronic respiratory failure.

Intervention in respiratory failure should be considered for patients with severe acidosis (pH < 7.26, H^+ > 55 nmol/L) and a rising CO_2 who fail to respond to supportive treatment with controlled oxygen therapy. In general, the indications for invasive mechanical ventilation are:

- persistent hypoxemia (PaO_2 < 5.3 kPa (40 mmHg)) despite maximum therapy
- worsening acute respiratory acidosis despite maximum therapy (pH < 7.25, H^+ > 55 nmol/L).

Other relative indications are:

- severe breathlessness with a respiratory frequency greater than 35 breaths/minute
- somnolence, impaired mental status
- inability to protect the airway
- inability to clear copious sputum
- respiratory arrest.

There is considerable debate over the appropriateness of invasive ventilation in end-stage COPD. However, mortality among COPD patients with respiratory failure is no greater than mortality among patients ventilated for non-COPD causes.

Factors that encourage the use of invasive intermittent positive-pressure ventilation (IPPV) include:

- demonstrable remediable reason for current decline, for example radiographic evidence of pneumonia or drug overdose
- first episode of respiratory failure
- acceptable quality of life, habitual level of activity.

Factors that discourage the use of invasive IPPV include:

- previously documented severe COPD in a patient who has been assessed and found to be unresponsive to relevant therapy
- poor quality of life – housebound despite maximum appropriate therapy
- severe comorbidities.

Age and the level of $PaCO_2$ are not a guide to the outcome of assisted ventilation in respiratory failure for COPD. A pH of less than 7.26 is associated with a higher mortality in acute exacerbations of COPD.

Non-invasive intermittent positive-pressure ventilation (NIPPV) has been shown in randomized controlled trials to be associated with fewer intubations, decreased mortality and shorter ICU admissions. The best time to start non-invasive ventilation is not established; however, a recent consensus statement from the American Association of Respiratory Care endorses the early use of NIPPV in exacerbations of COPD in the following circumstances:

- respiratory distress with moderate/severe dyspnea
- pH < 7.35 or $PaCO_2$ > 6 kPa (45 mmHg)
- respiratory rate of 25 breaths/minute or greater.

NIPPV is contraindicated in the presence of cardiovascular instability, craniofacial trauma or inability to protect the airways.

Hospital discharge and follow-up

There are no data indicating the optimal duration of hospitalization for acute exacerbations of COPD, but suggested discharge criteria are given in Table 8.5. Follow-up assessment 4–6 weeks after discharge from hospital is recommended (Table 8.6). The presence of hypoxemia

TABLE 8.5

Discharge criteria for patients with acute exacerbations of COPD

- Inhaled β-agonist therapy is required no more frequently than every 4 h
- Patient, if previously ambulatory, is able to walk across room
- Patient is able to eat and sleep without frequent disruption by dyspnea
- Patients has been clinically stable for 12–24 h
- Arterial blood gases have been stable for 12–24 h
- Patient (or home caregiver) fully understands correct use of medications
- Follow-up and home care arrangements have been completed
  (e.g. visiting nurse, oxygen delivery, meal provisions)
- Patient, family and physician are confident that patient can manage
  successfully

during an exacerbation of COPD should prompt rechecking of blood gases at discharge. If the patient remains hypoxemic, the need for long-term outpatient oxygen therapy should be assessed when the patient attains a stable state.

Recent randomized controlled trials have shown that 20–30% of patients hospitalized with acute exacerbations of COPD can be safely allowed home with supported discharge without adverse outcome.

TABLE 8.6

Follow-up assessment 4–6 weeks after discharge from hospital for acute exacerbations of COPD

- Assess ability to cope in usual environment
- Measure FEV_1
- Reassess inhaler technique
- Check patient's understanding of recommended treatment regimen
- Assess need for long-term oxygen therapy and/or home nebulizer
  (for patients with severe COPD)

FEV_1, forced expiratory volume in 1 second

Key points – acute exacerbations of COPD

- Acute exacerbations of COPD are common and place a huge burden on healthcare resources.
- The main etiologic factors are bacterial infection, respiratory viruses and air pollution.
- Treatment includes oxygen, increased bronchodilators, antibiotics, short-tem oral corticosteroids.
- Exacerbations can be prevented by inhaled corticosteroids and vaccination against influenza.
- Most exacerbations of COPD are managed at home, but those with suspected respiratory failure should be admitted to hospital.
- Non-invasive ventilation has been shown to reduce mortality in patients with acute-on-chronic respiratory failure.

Key references

Anthonisen NR, Manfreda J, Warren CPW et al. Antibiotic therapy in exacerbations of chronic obstructive pulmonary disease. *Ann Intern Med* 1987;106:196–204.

Cooper CB. Domiciliary oxygen therapy. In: Calverley PMA, Pride NB, eds. *Chronic Obstructive Pulmonary Disease*. London: Chapman & Hall, 1995:495–526.

Davies L, Angus RM, Calverley PMA. Oral corticosteroid in patients admitted to hospital with exacerbations of COPD: a prospective randomized trial. *Lancet* 1999;354:456–60.

Griffiths TL, Phillips CJ, Davies S et al. Cost-effectiveness of an outpatient multidisciplinary pulmonary rehabilitation programme. *Thorax* 2001;56:779–84.

MacNee W. Acute exacerbations of COPD. Consensus conference on management of chronic obstructive pulmonary disease. *J R Coll Phys Edinb*. 2002;32:1–46.

Medical Research Council Oxygen Working Party Report. Long-term domiciliary oxygen therapy in chronic carboxy cor pulmonale complicating chronic bronchitis and emphysema. *Lancet* 1981;1:681–6.

What the reviewers say:

This book is a little goldmine and is very good value for money

On *Fast Facts – Endometriosis, 2nd edn*, in *Medical Journal of Australia* 2004

concise and well written and accompanied by numerous excellent color illustrations... an excellent little book! Score: 100 - 5 Stars

On *Fast Facts – Sexual Dysfunction*
in *Doody's Health Sciences Review*, 2004

this small volume is pleasingly pithy, erudite and accessible, as well as being helpfully informative

On *Fast Facts – Bipolar Disorder, 2nd edn*, in *Medical Journal of Australia* 2004

a timely and accessible book...
a worthwhile and handy tool for medical students

On *Fast Facts – Dyspepsia*, in *Digestive and Liver Disease* 36, 2004

provides a lot of information in a concise and easily accessible format...
a practical guide to managing most lower respiratory tract infections

On *Fast Facts – Respiratory Tract Infection*,
in *Respiratory Care* 49(1), 2004

an invaluable guide to the latest thinking

On *Fast Facts – Irritable Bowel Syndrome*, in *Update*, 4 September 2003

a rapid guide to understanding dementia...
value for money and I would definitely recommend it

On *Fast Facts – Dementia*, in *South African Medical Journal* 93(10), 2003

excellent coverage of symptoms and diagnosis

On *Fast Facts – Dyspepsia*, in *Update*, 19 June, 2003

will likely be read cover to cover in just one or
two sittings by all who are fortunate enough
to obtain a copy

On *Fast Facts – Benign Prostatic Hyperplasia*, 4th edn, in *Doody's Health Sciences Review*, Dec 2002

explains the important facts and demonstrates
the levels of "good practice" that can be achieved

On *Fast Facts – Minor Surgery*,
in *Journal of the Royal Society for the Promotion of Health* 122(3), 2002

a splendid publication

On *Fast Facts – Sexually Transmitted Infections*, in *Journal of Antimicrobial Chemotherapy* 49, 2002

I would highly recommend it
without reservation... 5 stars!

On *Fast Facts – Psychiatry Highlights 2001–02*,
in *Doody's Health Sciences Review*, Sept 2002

I enthusiastically recommend this
stimulating, short book which should
be required reading for all clinicians

On *Fast Facts – Irritable Bowel Syndrome*, in *Gastroenterology* 120(6), 2001

***** outstanding

On *Fast Facts – HIV in Obstetrics and Gynecology*, in *Journal of Pelvic Surgery*, 2001

www.fastfacts.com

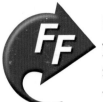

Imagine if every time you wanted to know something you knew where to look...

Over one million copies sold

- Written by world experts
- Concise and practical
- Up to date
- Designed for ease of reading and reference
- Copiously illustrated with useful photographs, diagrams and charts.

Our aim is to make *Fast Facts* the world's most respected medical handbook series. Feedback on how to make titles even more useful is always welcome (feedback@fastfacts.com).

More than 70 *Fast Facts* titles, including:

Asthma
Benign Gynecological Disease (second edition)
Benign Prostatic Hyperplasia (fifth edition)
Bipolar Disorder
Bladder Cancer
Bleeding Disorders
Brain Tumors
Breast Cancer (third edition)
Celiac Disease
Chronic Obstructive Pulmonary Disease
Colorectal Cancer (second edition)
Contraception (second edition)
Dementia
Depression (second edition)
Dyspepsia (second edition)
Eczema and Contact Dermatitis
Endometriosis (second edition)
Epilepsy (third edition)
Erectile Dysfunction (third edition)
Gynecological Oncology
Headaches (second edition)

Hyperlipidemia (third edition)
Hypertension (second edition)
Inflammatory Bowel Disease (second edition)
Irritable Bowel Syndrome (second edition)
Menopause (second edition)
Minor Surgery
Multiple Sclerosis (second edition)
Osteoporosis (fourth edition)
Parkinson's Disease
Prostate Cancer (fourth edition)
Psoriasis (second edition)
Respiratory Tract Infection (second edition)
Rheumatoid Arthritis
Schizophrenia (second edition)
Sexual Dysfunction
Sexually Transmitted Infections
Skin Cancer
Smoking Cessation
Soft Tissue Rheumatology
Thyroid Disorders
Urinary Stones

Orders

To order via the website, or to find regional distributors, please go to **www.fastfacts.com**

For telephone orders, please call +44 (0)1752 202301 (Europe), 1 800 247 6553 (USA, toll free) or +1 419 281 1802 (Americas)